M. J. DAVIES

Cardiovascular Pathology

OXFORD COLOUR ATLASES OF PATHOLOGY

OXFORD COLOUR ATLASES OF PATHOLOGY
GENERAL EDITOR: R. C. CURRAN, MD · FRCP · FRS (Edinburgh) · FRCPath

COLOUR ATLAS OF

Cardiovascular

Pathology

BY M. J. DAVIES, MD · FRCPath

British Heart Foundation Professor of Cardiovascular Pathology
St. George's Hospital Medical School, University of London

WITH 417 ILLUSTRATIONS IN COLOUR

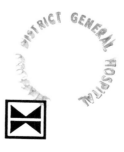

HARVEY MILLER PUBLISHERS
OXFORD UNIVERSITY PRESS

Originating Publisher HARVEY MILLER LTD
20 Marryat Road · London SW19 5BD · England

Published in conjunction with OXFORD UNIVERSITY PRESS
Walton Street · Oxford OX2 6DP

London · Glasgow · New York
Toronto · Melbourne · Auckland
Kuala Lumpur · Singapore · Hong Kong · Tokyo
Delhi · Bombay · Calcutta · Madras · Karachi
Nairobi · Dar es Salaam · Cape Town
and associates in Beirut · Ibadan · Mexico City · Nicosia

Published in the United States by
OXFORD UNIVERSITY PRESS · NEW YORK

British Library Cataloguing in Publication Data

Davies, M. J.
    Colour atlas of cardiovascular pathology.
    —(Oxford colour atlases of pathology; 4)
    1. Cardiovascular system—Diseases—Atlases
    I. Title
    616.1'0022'2   RC669

ISBN 0-19-921047-0

Illustrations originated by Schwitter AG · Basle · Switzerland
Text set by BSC Print Ltd · London SW18
Printed by Printing House Ljudska Pravica Ljubljana, Yugoslavia
Manufactured in Yugoslavia

Contents

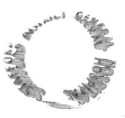

Preface

THE DEVELOPMENT of new techniques for imaging the heart has wrought radical changes in the field of cardiology. A close dialogue between the clinician and pathologist is essential for the interpretation of these images. This Atlas bridging, in word and picture, the traditional and the new techniques of cardiopathology, is directed primarily to the practising pathologist and pathologist-in-training, but should be of interest also to clinicians, cardiologists and cardiac surgeons. It covers the majority of cardiac conditions the pathologist is likely to encounter in his everyday practice, as well as more rare conditions.

For the morbid anatomist it is the advent of echocardiography which has been most significant. Modern echocardiography is not the preserve of sophisticated centres, but is carried out nowadays in every district general hospital. Echocardiography has made it possible to produce moving images of the structure of the living heart. The clinician's interest in morphology has thereby been reawakened, and he turns to the pathologist for explanation.

The clinician, however, examines the heart in planes determined by the requirement of echocardiographic access through windows in the chest wall, between boney structures. These planes are not those previously used by anatomists or pathologists, who dissect the heart by time-honoured methods, opening each chamber and valve in turn in the direction of the blood flow. Such methods, which long pre-dated echocardiography, owed little to function.

Cardiac pathology now has two objectives: that of the pathologist seeking detailed clinical correlation, examining the heart with the valves intact or transected in echocardiographic planes; and that used when carrying out routine autopsies to exclude cardiac disease. The two procedures need not be, and should not be mutually exclusive, and both approaches are adopted here, as appropriate: the normal structure of the heart is described in Chapter 1 using both procedures.

New techniques have induced a comparable revolution in relation to the assessment of coronary disease by pathologists. Selective angiography of the coronary arteries in life is now commonplace, and pathologists must be prepared to be more precise about the exact location and degree of areas of stenosis.

Cardiac pathology is less dependent on histology than is, for example, hepatic pathology or neuropathology. This largely reflects the limited morphological responses of the myocardium to damage. However, there are some specific histological responses and appearances which should be recognized by pathologists and understood by clinicians, and these are shown in this Atlas.

Acquired heart disease is covered in Chapters 3-9, and includes valve disease, infective endocarditis, cardiomyopathies, ischemic heart disease and cardiac tumours.

In the past, morphological studies of the coronary arteries in ischemic heart disease, of necessity, lacked functional correlates with regard to the blood flow. This situation has now changed, with the advent of selective coronary arteriography as a routine procedure in all forms of acute and chronic ischemic heart disease. Such studies now emphasize the variable or 'dynamic' nature of many obstructive lesions which could not have been predicted by a post mortem study. The variation in the degree of obstruction is due either to lysis of thrombosis, or to alterations in medial muscle tone. This work has necessitated a reappraisal of the role of spasm and thrombosis with regard to atheroma in the coronary arteries, and this aspect is stressed in Chapter 6. Here, too, the considerable advances in the understanding of the biochemical and structural consequences of ischemia in dog myocardium are discussed and illustrated, and the close analogy between this experimental model and human ischemic damage is emphasized.

Another significant change has been in valve disease in Western countries due to the decline of rheumatic fever, and in the non-rheumatic causes of stenosis and incompetence dealt with in Chapters 3 and 4. At the same time chronic rheumatic valve disease is also fully covered here, reflecting the continuing importance of this disease in the Third World. Bacterial endocarditis has changed largely due to the new ways in which infection can be introduced following cardiac surgery or drug addiction, and these aspects are covered in Chapter 5, while Chapter 7 deals with the morphological expressions of the different forms of cardiomyopathy. Here the functional aspects of each are stressed.

Congenital heart disease presents in a myriad of forms, many of which are very rare; and although more specialized publications provide a comprehensive guide to these conditions, Chapter 10 of this Atlas explains and illustrates the principal forms likely to be encountered.

Especially useful will be the illustrations in Chapter 11 devoted to Cardiac surgery. Cardiac surgery is now common, and pathologists must have a modicum of knowledge concerning the fate of vein grafts and the commonly used valve prostheses. Individual pathologists will not carry out large numbers of autopsies in this field, and for them this part of the Atlas will be of particular importance.

The photographs have all been taken from my own collection with the exception of the congenital abnormalities, which are from museum specimens.

I acknowledge with thanks the help of Ms Jane Fallows, who drew the diagrams, and Mrs P. McKinnon who typed the manuscript.

Atlas of
Cardiovascular Pathology

CHAPTER 1

Normal Structure
of the Heart

ROUTINE DISSECTION
OF THE HEART
(1.1 – 1.9)

The routine technique used by most pathologists to display the heart is to open each chamber and valve in a sequence which follows the direction of blood flow and begins at the opening of the inferior vena cava into the right atrium. The technique is honoured by time and easy to learn, since it merely requires an ability to recognize the anatomical landmarks of each chamber. Most illustrations of cardiac pathology in standard text books are of hearts displayed in this manner. For these reasons and also for the fact that the technique is used by most pathologists in routine autopsy work to exclude a cardiac abnormality, complete familiarity with anatomy so displayed is required of the pathologist in training.

The conventional dissection technique is limited, however, because it bears little relation to modern cardiology practice and it approaches the heart in a manner likely to obscure rather than illustrate function. Valve function, for example, cannot be appreciated once the ring has been opened. Clinical echocardiography allows both static and moving images to be made in two dimensional planes. The planes are governed by the windows in the chest wall through which the echo beam can be directed, so they cannot be altered. Thus, the cardiologist now examines the heart in a series of transections in different planes. These can be easily reproduced in the post-mortem room and they provide elegant clinico-pathological correlation clearly understood by clinicians.

The pathologist at the present time, therefore, should be prepared to dissect the heart in a manner most appropriate to the clinician's needs and to the questions asked of the post-mortem examination. This will require an ability to recognize the anatomical landmarks of the opened chambers and valves as well as the three most common echocardiographic planes: short axis, long axis and apical four chamber. In addition, knowledge of the normal function of the aortic and mitral valve and of coronary artery anatomy is required.

When using the conventional dissection technique (1.1-1.9), the right atrium is opened by a cut from the orifice of the inferior vena cava into the atrial appendage, allowing inspection of the atrial septum. The main landmark is an oval depression marking the site of the fossa ovalis, posterior and inferior to which lies the opening of the coronary sinus. The right ventricle is initially opened by a lateral incision from the atrium through the tricuspid valve into the apex of the right ventricle. The cut is then continued up through the anterior wall of the outflow tract and pulmonary valve into the main pulmonary artery. The opened tricuspid valve rarely appears to have three well-defined cusps; the most constant feature is the large anterior cusp suspended between the inflow and outflow portions of the right ventricle. The tricuspid and pulmonary valves are not in continuity since there is a mass of muscle, the supraventricular crest, separating the inflow and outflow portions of the right ventricle.

The left atrium is a featureless chamber, apart from the opening of the appendage. The left ventricle is opened by a cut through the lateral margin of the mitral valve ring, thus displaying the inflow tract and the two cusps of the mitral valve. The anterior cusp is different in shape from the posterior, as well as being larger and thicker. Chordae from both the antero-lateral and postero-medial papillary muscles in the left ventricle join each cusp. Next, the outflow tract of the left ventricle is opened either through the anterior wall of the ventricle or through the anterior cusp of the mitral valve itself. The cut is continued up through the aortic valve into the aorta. The left side of the interventricular septum is relatively smooth, while the remainder of the ventricular cavity, particularly the apical portion, is trabeculated. The aortic valve normally has three cusps, although in around 1% of individuals it has only two (bicuspid aortic valve). The right and left coronary artery orifices open from the aortic sinuses, just above the ridge which marks the junction of the aortic valve ring with the aorta.

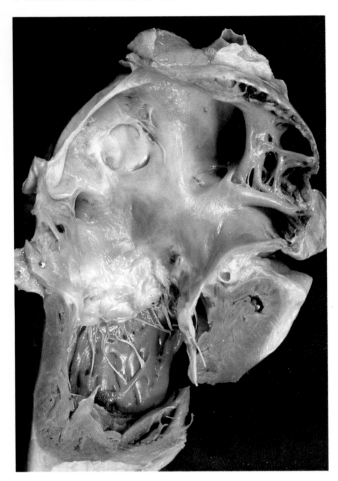

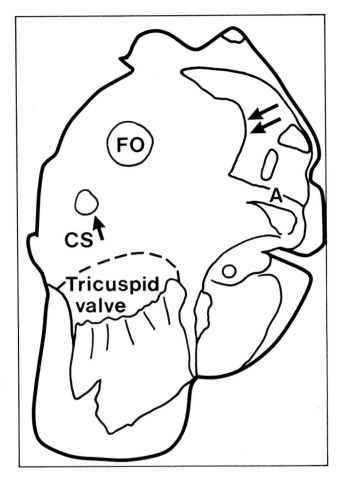

1.1 Right atrium

1.1 Anatomical features of the right atrium (with diagram). The interatrial septum viewed after opening the right atrium by a cut running from the inferior vena cava to the tip of the atrial appendage. The foramen ovale (FO) is the round depression in the centre of the septum. The coronary sinus (arrow) is the small orifice, often partially covered by a residual valve-like structure posterior and inferior to the foramen ovale. A prominent ridge (double arrow), the crista terminalis, surrounds the superior vena caval orifice and separates the trabeculated muscle of the appendage (A) from the smoother atrial septum. The superior vena cava is best left intact to preserve the sinus node for later histological examination if required. The sinus node lies in the junction of the superior vena cava and atrium just at the crest of the atrial appendage.

1.2 The interatrial septum viewed from the right side by transillumination. Two areas, which consist only of thin fibrous tissue, transmit the light. The larger is the foramen ovale, an oval or round area within the muscular atrial septum. The floor of the oval foramen is formed by a fibrous septum which has fused to the rim of the defect on the left side. The triangular bright area below and anterior to the foramen ovale is the membranous interventricular septum. The arrows mark the site of the sinus node at the crest of the atrial appendage and the atrioventricular node which lies anterior to the coronary sinus posterior to the membranous septum and just above the insertion of the septal cusp of the tricuspid valve. The septal cusp of the tricuspid valve (S) crosses the membranous portion of the ventricular septum. The membranous septum is thus divided into a portion above the insertion of the valve cusp which separates the atria; and an inferior portion which separates right and left ventricles.

1.3 Probe patency of the atrial septum. The atrial septum is viewed from the right. The picture shows a heart in which it has been possible to pass a probe through the foramen ovale anteriorly where the floor has not fully fused to the rim of the opening in the septum. Some degree of such probe patency can be found in approximately 20% of adult hearts.

1.4 Chiari Net in the right atrium. In the fetal heart there is a valve at the opening of the inferior vena cava. Remnants often persist into adult life as strands or nets of fibrous tissue around the opening of the coronary sinus and inferior vena cava. Strands may cross the cavity of the atrium. They have no functional or pathological significance.

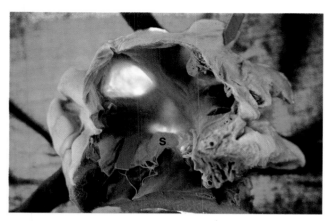

1.2 Interatrial septum: transilluminated

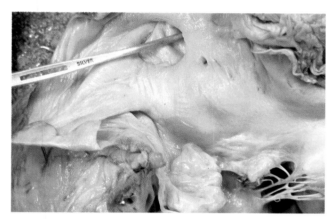

1.3 Probe patency

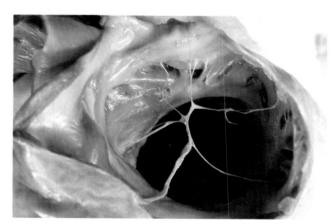

1.4 Chiari net

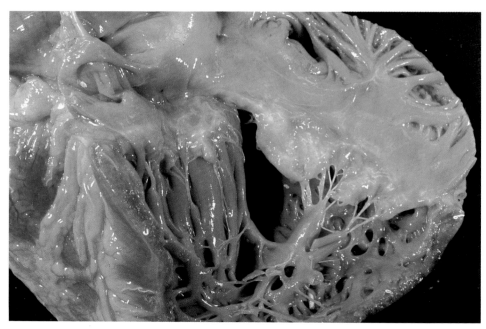

1.5 Landmarks of the right ventricle

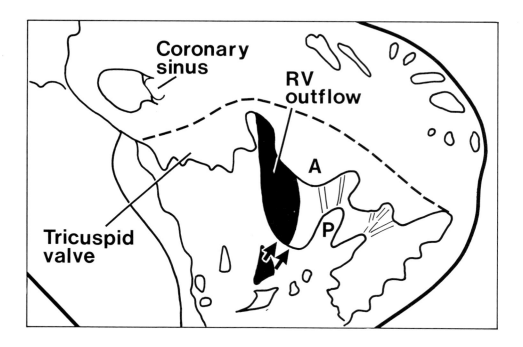

1.5 Anatomical landmarks of the right ventricle (with diagram). The right ventricle has been opened down its sharp lateral margin to display the tricuspid valve and right side of the interventricular septum. The anterior cusp of the tricuspid valve (A) separates the inflow portion of the right ventricle from the outflow tract. The axes of the inflow and outflow tracts thus are at right angles. The moderator band (double arrow) is a ridge of muscle low on the septum which carries the right bundle branch to the anterior wall of the ventricle. Most of the ventricle, particularly the apical portion, is heavily trabeculated. The papillary muscles are very variable in anatomy; the most constant is the anterior shown here (P), to which the moderator band joins.

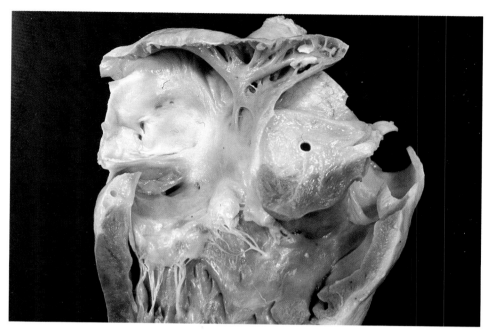

1.6 Right ventricle: inflow and outflow

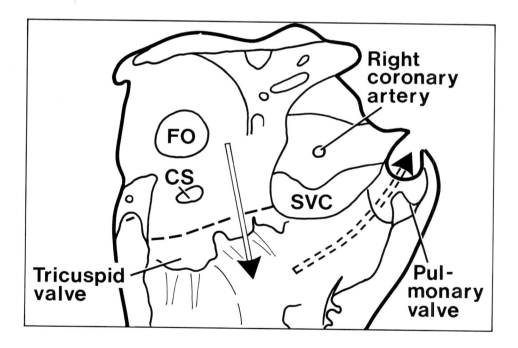

1.6 Inflow and outflow portions of the right ventricle (with diagram). The atrial and ventricular septum are viewed from the right side after removing the lateral wall of the ventricle. The inflow portion of the ventricle is marked by an arrow. The outflow track (dotted arrow) is at right angles. The inflow and outflow tracts are separated by a wedge of muscle, the supraventricular crest (SVC). Thus, the tricuspid valve does not have direct continuity with the pulmonary valve.

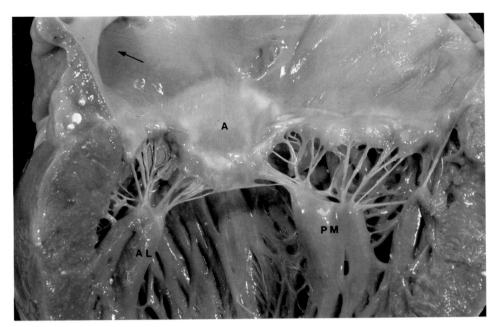

1.7 Mitral valve

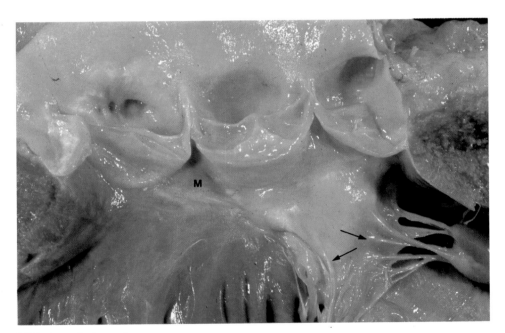

1.8 Left ventricular outflow

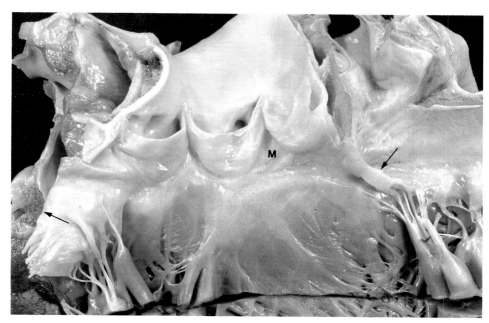

1.9 Left ventricular outflow

1.7 Anatomical features of the mitral valve and inflow portion of the left ventricle.
The left atrium and ventricle are displayed by a cut through the lateral aspect of the mitral valve ring. The left atrium is featureless apart from the opening of the appendage (arrow). The anterior cusp of the mitral valve (A) is semi-circular in shape with chordae inserted into the lateral aspects of its free edge. The shape of the posterior cusp is oblong, with one long edge attached to the valve ring, while from the other long free edge chordae insert into the papillary muscles. The papillary muscles are grouped into anterior-lateral (AL) and posterior-medial (PM) groups. They may be single structures or be subdivided into smaller heads. The lateral and medial commissures are marked by special chordae which break up into a fan of insertions into each cusp, shown against a blue background.

1.8 The anatomical features of the left ventricular outflow.
The left ventricular outflow has been opened by a cut running up the anterior wall of the ventricle. This allows the anterior cusp of the mitral valve to be retained intact, hinged to the anterior wall of the ventricle. This technique demonstrates the importance of the anterior cusp in separating the inflow and outflow portions of the left ventricle. The chordae to the anterior cusp of the mitral valve are inserted into a 'rough zone' (arrows) on the ventricular, i.e. outflow side. Lipid deposition beneath the endocardium in this high-pressure side of the cusp is very common but of no clinical importance. The membranous portion of the interventricular septum (M) is the triangular area just beneath the aortic valve and anterior to the junction of the base of the anterior cusp of the mitral valve with the aortic valve. The continuity between the anterior cusp of the mitral valve and the aortic valve is shown.

1.9 Anatomical features of the left ventricular outflow.
In contrast to **1.8** the left ventricular outflow has been opened through the anterior cusp of the mitral valve. The advantages of this method of dissection are in the ease with which the cut is made and the good display of the aortic valve and the ventricular cavity. The anterior cusp of the mitral valve is divided into two (arrows). The membranous interventricular septum (M) is well displayed and since the septum is flattened in fixation it is easy to take histological blocks through this area to study the conduction system. The disadvantages are the total destruction of the mitral valve anatomy and the fact that any display of the normal relations of the outflow tract to the mitral valve is masked. This artificial destruction of the anatomical relations produces a specimen which is incomprehensible to clinicians.

DISSECTION OF THE HEART
IN ECHOCARDIOGRAPHIC PLANES
(1.10 – 1.15)

Dissection of the heart in echocardiographic planes is remarkably simple: all that is needed is a long sharp knife to bisect the specimen and knowledge of where to make the cuts. If the heart is bisected in the longitudinal axis through the anterior cusp of the mitral valve and the aortic valve, the plane is created which is used in both M mode and the two dimensional (2D) long axis echocardiographic view. The plane bisects the left ventricle through both its inflow and outflow tracts, thus demonstrating the anatomy of both as well as that of the aortic and mitral valves. This plane is also used to obtain measurements of the interventricular septum and posterior wall of the left ventricle, as well as the size of aortic root and left atrium. Measurements made by these means in life closely correlate with the same measurements made in the postmortem room. The ability to draw and think in terms of the normal anatomy of this plane is crucial to pathologists who wish to understand modern cardiology.

Transverse slices across the short axis of the ventricles in a post-mortem specimen equate very closely with the short axis echocardiography planes. For pathologists the most useful is a one-centimetre thick slice taken at mid septal level, i.e. half-way between the apex of the ventricles and atrioventricular groove. Such a slice demonstrates the chamber sizes and wall thickness of both ventricles, and all can be measured. The distribution of myocardial infarction and scarring can also be correlated with the coronary artery anatomy. These transverse slices give a far better impression of the regional distribution of lesions, i.e. anterior, lateral, posterior or septal in the myocardium than the conventional dissection technique.

The third commonly used plane in clinical medicine, the apical four-chamber view, is again in the long axis but at 90 degrees to that previously described. It displays all four chambers and their relation to each other, as well as the atrial and ventricular septae. It is of great use in congenital heart lesions, but less so in adults.

The short and long axis views described can all be made by simply bisecting the intact heart, fresh or fixed, with a long sharp knife. In practice, a short axis cut at mid septal level, followed by a long axis on the upper half of the specimen, is ideal. Provided the coronary arteries and examined and the aortic and mitral valves are inspected before such cuts are made, all eventualities are covered. By clinical convention, clinical echocardiograms are displayed with the posterior wall downward and ventricular apex pointing to the left.

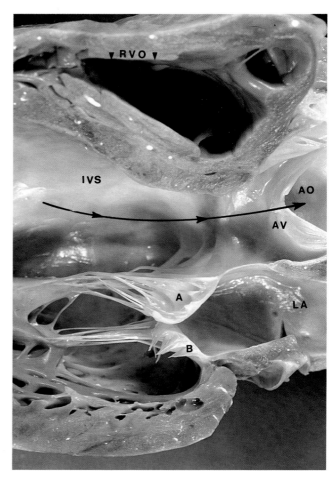

1.10 Heart: long axis

1.10 Long axis view of the heart. This plane is portrayed by echocardiographic convention with the apex toward the left and the anterior surface of the heart upward, i.e. as if the heart was in situ in a supine patient. The left atrium (LA) lies immediately adjacent and behind the aorta (AO). The atrium opens into the inflow portion of the left ventricle, between the papillary muscles and guarded by the cusps of the mitral valve, anterior (A) and posterior (B). Below the papillary muscles is the apical portion of the left ventricular cavity. A solid curved arrow indicates the outflow path of the left ventricle toward and through the aortic valve into the aorta. Below the aortic valve (AV), the outflow is bounded on one side by the anterior cusp of the mitral valve and on the other by the interventricular septum (IVS). Thus the anterior cusp of the mitral valve separates the inflow and outflow portions of the left ventricle. The other key fact is that the anterior cusp of the mitral valve actually inserts into the aortic valve, i.e. there is aortic-mitral continuity. The outflow tract of the right ventricle (RVO) lies anterior to that of the left, which is crossed at right angles.

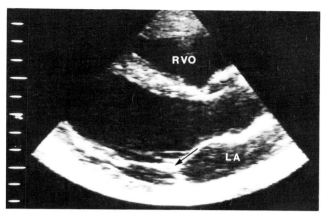

1.11a Long axis: mitral valve closed

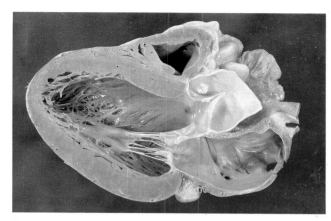

1.12 Long axis: M mode echo

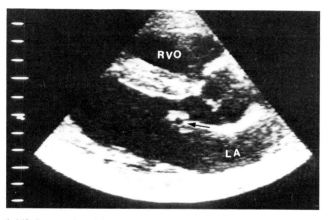

1.11b Long axis: mitral valve open

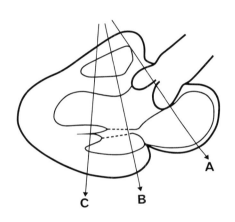

1.11a and b   2D echocardiogram in the long axis view. The echo beam is fan shaped, and the apex of the left ventricle is often not displayed. The anatomy of the left ventricular outflow is shown in exactly the plane illustrated in **1.10.** The right ventricular outflow (RVO) is at the apex of the fan, that is anterior in the patient. The left atrium (LA) is posterior behind the aorta. The mitral valve (arrow) is shown in **a** in the closed position; in **b** the mitral valve is shown open. In life the actual movement of the mitral cusps can be watched on the screen.

1.12   M mode echocardiography and the long axis of the heart (with diagram). In M mode echocardiography a pencil beam of ultrasound is aimed across the long axis, reflecting back from the structures to produce an image. If the beam is angled across the aortic root (A), its dimensions can be measured. Such a beam also traverses the left atrium, making measurement possible. Angling the beam low at (B) allows the movement of the anterior and posterior cusps of the mitral valve to be followed as they open and close. At this level, the width of the left ventricular outflow, i.e. between interventricular septum and anterior cusp, can also be measured. Lower still the beam traverses the ventricular cavity (C) which can be measured in systole and diastole.

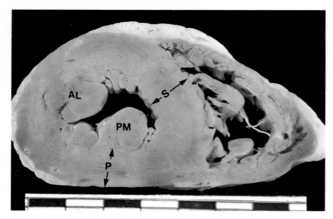

1.13 Short axis: left ventricle

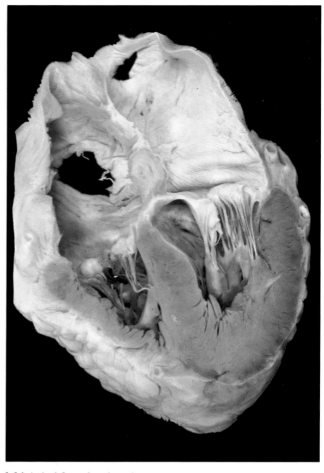

1.14 Apical four-chamber view

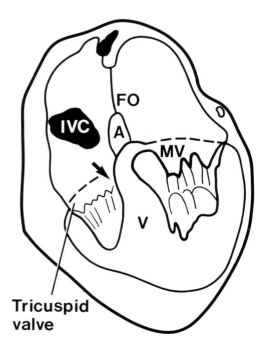

1.13 Short axis transection of the left ventricle. A transverse slice across both ventricles at mid-septal level. The left ventricle is a ring of muscle, on one side of which is attached the right ventricle, a triangular structure. There are two main papillary muscles in the left ventricle: antero-lateral (AL) and postero-medial (PM). The dimensions of the left ventricle which are usually measured are the septal thickness (S), the posterior wall thickness (P), excluding the papillary muscles, and the mean of two diameters of the left ventricular cavity. The posterior wall of the left ventricle can be identified because it is flatter and straighter than the curved anterior wall. Sections taken above the papillary muscles will also show that the right ventricular outflow begins to curve across in front of and anterior to the left ventricle. A short axis echocardiogram displays an identical picture.

1.14 Apical four-chamber view of the heart (with diagram). In a heart bisected in this plane all four cardiac chambers are shown. The atrial (A) and ventricular (V) septae are both seen 'end-on' and are not quite in line; the atrial septum normally lies to the left. The tricuspid valve (arrow) is inserted lower on the septum than the mitral (MV), which aids identification in complex congenital abnormalities. In the atrial septum the fibrous sheet forming the foramen ovale (FO) is shown. The orifice of the inferior vena cava (IVC) is seen 'en face'.

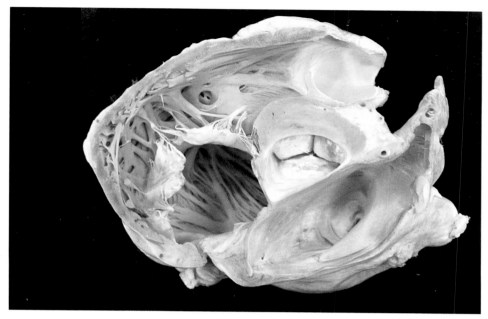

1.15 Short axis

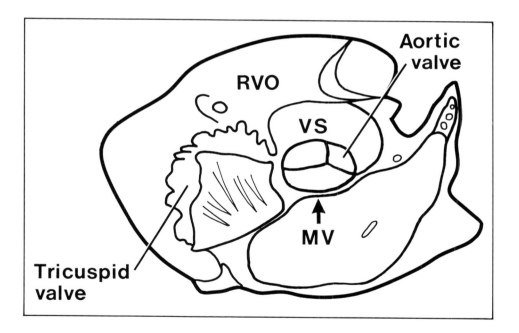

1.15 Short axis transection of the heart just below the aortic valve (with diagram). In this view, the aortic valve can be seen 'end-on' from below. In life it is a good view to assess stenosis. The orifice of the aortic valve at the sub-valve level is ringed by the base of the anterior cusp of the mitral valve and the upper ventricular septum. In this plane the whole outflow tract of the right ventricle (RVO) is seen in its long axis.

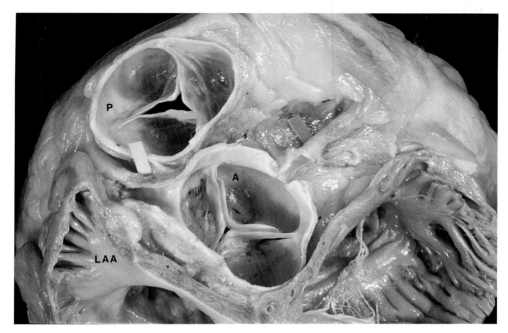

1.16 Aortic root

THE CORONARY ARTERIES
AND AORTIC ROOT
(1.16 – 1.20)

The normal anatomical arrangement is for a coronary artery to arise from each of the anterior-facing aortic sinuses of Valsalva, which are therefore called the right and left coronary sinuses. The pulmonary trunk lies in front of the aorta and the non-coronary sinus of the aorta faces directly posteriorly.

The distribution of the coronary arteries to the myocardium is very variable in its detail, but certain broad principles apply to virtually every human heart. The main left coronary artery gives rise to the left anterior descending coronary artery, which runs on the anterior surface of the heart in the interventricular groove. This artery and its branches supply between 40% and 60% of the left ventricular muscle mass on the anterior and lateral aspects of the heart, as well as sending perforating vessels into the anterior two-thirds of the interventricular septum. The level in the ventricle at which the artery divides into smaller vessels is very variable, as is the degree to which the apex of the ventricle is supplied. In extreme cases the artery turns around the apex to run upward for a short distance on the posterior wall. The other major branch of the left coronary artery is the circumflex artery, which runs in the left atrioventricular groove of the heart to supply, via marginal branches, the myocardium of the lateral wall of the left ventricle. The right coronary artery runs in the right atrioventricular groove to reach the

posterior wall of the heart, where it turns downward to become the posterior descending coronary artery in the posterior interventricular groove. The right coronary artery supplies the right ventricular myocardium, the posterior third of the interventricular septum and the posterior wall of the left ventricle. In any individual heart, the right coronary and the left circumflex arteries are inversely related in size, and in the proportion of left ventricular muscle that is supplied.

The term 'dominance' is used in two ways. One use is to indicate which artery is giving origin to the posterior descending branch. In approximately two-thirds of individuals it is the right, as described above. In 30% of individuals (left-dominant) the left circumflex gives rise to the posterior descending artery. The other use of the word 'dominance' is not absolute but relative. It concerns whether the greater amount of the posterior wall of the left ventricular myocardium is supplied by the right or the left coronary artery. Thus it is possible for a heart to be right-dominant by the first definition but left-dominant by the second.

The atrial blood supply is highly variable; the sinus node is supplied by a vessel which may arise from either right or left coronary artery and which ultimately forms a ring around the root of the superior vena cava. The atrioventricular nodal artery always arises from the origin of the posterior descending coronary artery. The veins of the myocardium run toward a large vein, the coronary sinus, on the posterior atrioventricular groove which opens into the right atrium at the coronary sinus. There are rich lymphatics in the myocardium, but as yet no pathological process has been proven to involve these in human disease.

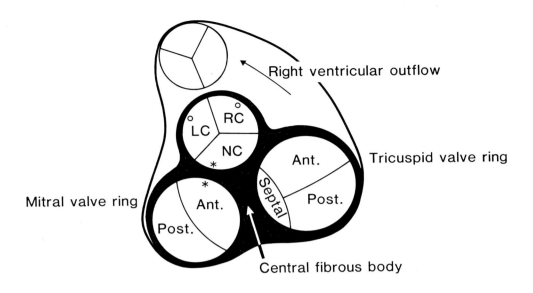

1.16a Fibrous skeleton of the heart and cusp nomenclature

1.16   Anatomy of the aortic root. The relation of the
pulmonary artery to the aorta, viewed from above after
removing the roof of the atria. The pulmonary trunk (P)
lies anteriorly and to the left; the aorta (A) is posterior and
to the right. From each of the two anterior-facing aortic
sinuses a coronary artery arises. The left coronary artery
is marked yellow, the right red. The logical nomenclature
of the sinuses is thus right, left and non-coronary. The
main left coronary artery lies between the pulmonary
trunk and the left atrial appendage (LAA).

**1.16a   Diagrammatic representation of the fibrous
skeleton of the heart and cusp nomenclature.** The
fibrous skeleton (black) supports the atrioventricular
valves and anchors them to the aortic valve and ventricular
muscle masses. The pulmonary valve is not directly
attached. Both atrioventricular valve annuli are continuous rings of connective tissue, conjoined at their
medial aspects to form a large mass which is known as the
central fibrous body. The aortic valve ring is attached to
the anterior and superior aspect of the central fibrous
body. There is thus continuity (*–*) between the attachment of the anterior cusp of the mitral valve and the
non-coronary cusp of the aortic valve. The nomenclature
of the aortic cusps and sinuses is non-coronary (NC)
facing posteriorly, left coronary (LC) and right coronary
(RC) facing left and right respectively, each giving rise to
a coronary artery. The potential sites of rupture of the rare
congenital aneurysms of the sinuses can be worked out
from the diagram. For example, the right sinus can rupture
into the right ventricular outflow, the non-coronary sinus
into the right or the left atrium.

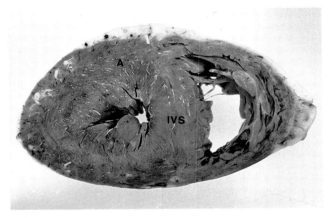

1.17 Myocardial blood supply

1.17   Myocardial blood supply. A transverse slice
across the right and left ventricles, corresponding to a
short axis echocardiogram. The coronary arteries have
been injected with different-coloured media. The left
anterior descending artery (yellow) supplies the anterior
(A) and lateral walls of the left ventricle and the bulk of
the muscular interventricular septum (IVS). The circumflex artery (blue) supplies a small area of the lateral
wall, while the right coronary artery (red) supplies the
posterior wall of the left ventricle including the postero-
medial muscle, some of the interventricular septum and
the whole of the right ventricle.

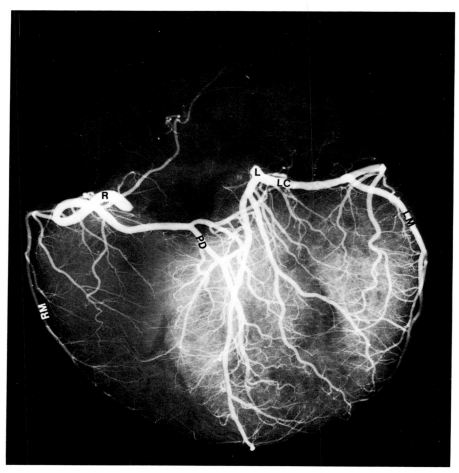

1.18 Right dominance

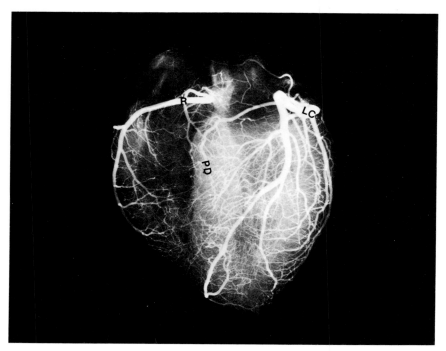

1.19 Left dominance

1.18 Normal coronary anatomy: right-dominance.
Post-mortem angiogram in an anterior-posterior view of a normal heart. The right coronary artery (R) passes around the right atrio-ventricular groove, supplying a marginal branch (RM) to the right ventricle. It then continues onto the posterior wall of the heart, becoming the posterior descending artery (PD), and finally passes across to supply a small part of the posterior wall of the left ventricle. The main left coronary artery (L) divides into the left anterior descending (LAD) and left circumflex (LC) arteries. The former has several major divisions supplying the anterior wall of the left ventricle. The left circumflex artery forms a left marginal branch (LM) to the lateral wall of the left ventricle. This heart is right-dominant, i.e. the right coronary artery supplies the posterior descending branch and continues on to supply the posterior wall of the left ventricle. The atrial artery supplying the sinus node (arrow) arises from the first part of the right coronary artery.

1.19 Normal coronary anatomy: left-dominance.
Post-mortem angiogram in an anterior-posterior view of a normal heart. The right coronary artery (R) supplies a right marginal but does not continue on to the posterior wall. The left circumflex artery (LC) passes round the left atrioventricular groove to form the posterior descending artery (PD). The main atrial artery which also supplies the sinus node artery (arrow) rises from the left circumflex artery.

1.20 Post-mortem angiogram of the isolated inter-atrial and interventricular septa. The foramen ovale and membranous septum are avascular and radiolucent. The left anterior descending artery (LAD) send numerous perforating vessels into the septum to meet other perforators from the posterior descending artery (PD). The anterior are longer than the posterior perforating branches. The anterior and posterior descending arteries meet at the apex of the septum. The anterior artery may turn the apex to pass up the posterior wall for a short distance in many hearts. The artery to the atrioventricular node (arrow) is the first perforating branch from the posterior descending artery and can be seen to run in the atria until it reaches the membranous septum. At this point it turns down to perforate the central fibrous body and reach the upper interventricular septum.

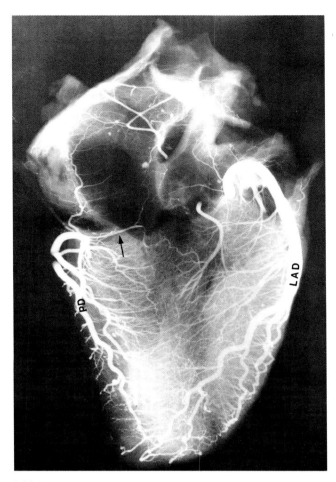

1.20 Interatrial and interventricular blood supply

MICROSTRUCTURE OF THE MYOCARDIUM (1.21 – 1.27)

The myocardium is not a syncytium. Individual cardiac muscle cells are essentially oblong in shape, but they do have lateral projections which interdigitate with those of their neighbours. The membranes of the short sides of the cells are fused at tight junctions thought to be important in the propagation of electrical impulses. These end-to-end junctions are known as intercalated discs.

There are complex arrangements of muscle layers, particularly in the left ventricle, and in any histological section there are myocardial cells cut in either the long or short axis. The right ventricular myocardium is always less orderly in arrangement and tends to show increasing fatty infiltration with age. The atrial muscle is also more haphazardly arranged and is infiltrated by adipose tissue particularly in hearts from subjects of Western communities. Between the myocardial cells is an anastomosing mesh of capillaries, so rich as to provide a vessel adjacent to every muscle fibre. The interstitial space contains a fine supporting stroma of collagen and related fibroblasts as well as numerous sympathetic and parasympathetic nerves. The interstitial space also contains a mixture of other cells, including mast cells, myofibroblasts, histiocytes and Anitschkow cells. The last is regarded as a modified fibroblast and may be recognized by a central bar of chromatin in the nucleus. It can be found in most infant and young hearts and is not in itself pathological.

The ultrastructural appearances of myocardial cells show the whole cell to be packed with regularly arranged myofibrils and to contain numerous mitochondria. The membranes of adjacent cells are fused tightly at the intercalated discs. In the perinuclear zone granules including lipofuscin are present. Within atrial muscle cells there are specific granules recently recognized to be the likely source of a diuretic hormone released following stretching and dilation of the atria.

1.21, 1.22   Histological appearances of normal myocardium: longitudinal section. Normal human myocardium cut in a plane longitudinal to the direction of the muscle fibres. The cell junctions at the intercalated discs are not identifiable in standard 6-8μm sections stained by hematoxylin and eosin, but they can be identified in phosphotungstic acid hematoxylin-stained (PTAH) sections. The myocardial cells in post-mortem material often separate through the intercalated discs (arrow). The PTAH section, however, shows that intercalated discs are more numerous than such separations suggest. Very short intercalated disc-to-disc distances are found in the lateral projections of myocardial cells. Each myocardial cell contains centrally placed nuclei, in the perinuclear zone brown lipofuscin granules are usually present. Between each muscle fibre is a capillary embedded in fine connective tissue, but these vessels are not easily identified in conventional sections.
1.21 x375 Hematoxylin and eosin.
1.22 x375 Phosphotungstic acid hematoxylin.

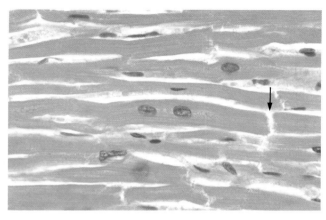

1.21 Normal myocardium

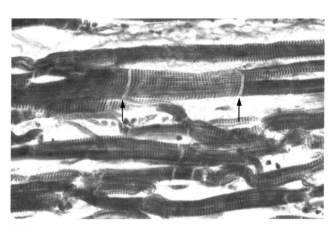

1.22 Normal myocardium

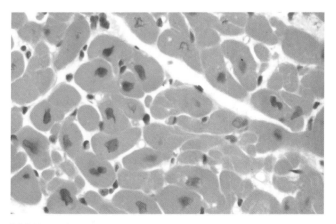

1.23 Normal myocardium

1.23   Normal myocardium: transverse histological section. Normal human left ventricular myocardium with the fibres cut in transverse section. Some fibres are cut in the plane of the nuclei; others have no nuclei visible. The nuclei in the interstitial spaces belong either to endothelial or to connective tissue cells.
x375 Hematoxylin and eosin.

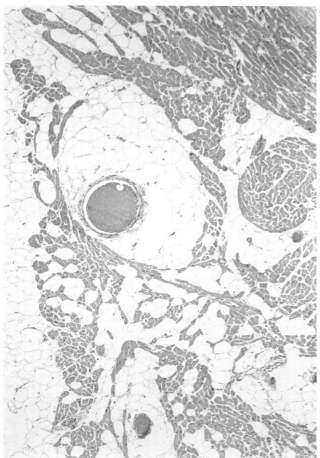

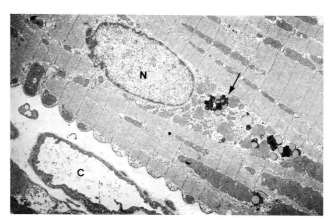

1.25 Ultrastructure of myocardium

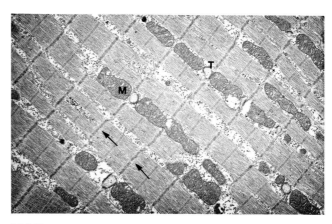

1.26 Ultrastructure of myocardium

1.24 Normal right ventricular myocardium

1.24 Normal human right ventricular myocardium. Right ventricular myocardium with considerable infiltration of adipose tissue between irregularly arranged myocardial cells.
x25 Hematoxylin and eosin.

1.25, 1.26, 1.27 Ultrastructure of normal myocardium. Electron microscopic sections of normal myocardium as seen in longitudinal section. **1.25** shows that adjacent to the nucleus (N) the perinuclear zone contains electron-dense granules of lipofuschin (arrow). In the interstitial space adjacent to the muscle cell is a capillary (C). In **1.26** the cytoplasm of the myocardial muscle cell is seen to be packed with dense regular arrays of thick and thin filaments or myofibrils; Z lines (arrows) are the dark electron-dense material to which the thick filaments are attached. The plasma membrane dips into the cell as the transverse tubules at each Z line. The transverse tubules (T), which connect to the external environment, abut onto another tubular system running internally through to the cell. Numerous mitochondria (M) are packed between the myofibrils. In **1.27** the intercalated discs (arrows) form step-like junctions across the short axis at the end of each cell. On the longitudinal edge of the steps the cell membranes fuse as tight junctions.

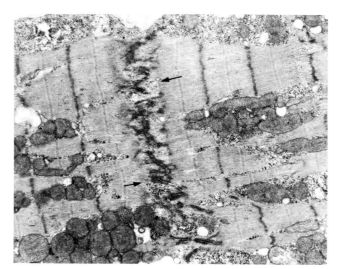

1.27 Ultrastructure of myocardium

CHAPTER 2

The Pathology
of Cardiac Failure

A simple working definition of cardiac failure for pathologists is the condition arising when contractile function of the heart is impaired to the point at which salt and water retention by the kidney has occurred in life.

The heart fails as a consequence of an increase in the workload on the ventricular muscle. This increase in workload may result from an increased volume of blood being pumped, as for example in aortic regurgitation or in congenital heart disease with left to right shunting. In these instances, the heart has to achieve a greater stroke volume than a normal heart to produce the same effective forward output of blood. Alternatively, the heart may have to eject blood against an increased pressure load, for example in aortic valve stenosis. Clinically and physiologically, these two forms of increased volume and pressure workload roughly equate to pre- and after-load and have different morphological effects on the ventricle.

Working against increased pressure leads to increase in the muscle mass of the affected ventricle, but a cavity of normal size is retained and hence the ventricular wall thickness is markedly increased. In volume overload the ventricular cavity enlarges, and therefore, despite an increase in muscle mass equivalent to that in pressure overload, the wall thickness is not greatly increased and may even be diminished. At first, volume or pressure overload usually affects only one ventricle. But while for simplicity the ventricles can be regarded as separate pumps, in heart failure salt and water retention leads to an increased blood volume and ultimately both ventricles will fail.

The pathologist endeavours to judge the effect of chronic overload on the heart by measuring hypertrophy of the myocardium. The parameter most widely used is total heart weight. This measurement does correlate directly with isolated left ventricular mass but gives no indication of right ventricular mass, since the latter forms a very small proportion of the total heart weight. Wall thickness, while measured in many post-mortem reports, gives no indication of ventricular weight since it depends more on cavity size than on muscle mass.

The technique which does give accurate data is the measurement of isolated ventricular muscle weights by the Fulton method (Appendix 3). Here, each ventricle is weighed separately after removing the pericardial fat and atria. The interventricular septum is regarded as functionally belonging to the left ventricle.

At a histological level the myocardial responses to pressure and volume overload are also different. In myocardial hypertrophy, individual muscle fibres increase in size and the nuclei become large and hyperchromatic due to tetraploidy. The number of muscle cells is not thought to increase, but the total amount of muscle DNA does rise. In pressure overload, individual muscle fibres become broader and the mean diameter, measured in cross-section, rises. In volume overload, similar nuclear changes occur but the mean muscle diameter shows only minimal increase, or even a reduction. This suggests an increase in muscle fibre length. Both forms of hypertrophy are associated with an increase in interstitial fibrous tissue. The stromal increase is more prominent in pressure overload, particularly in the subendocardial myocardium. No definite histological parameter marks the transition from compensatory hypertrophy to a 'failed' myocardium, although it does appear that much of the increase in ventricular mass in the later stages of hypertrophy is in fact stromal connective tissue and thus of no functional value.

Cardiac failure can also develop in ischemic damage to the myocardium or in cardiomyopathies. The only difference is that failure results from increased volume and pressure load on the proportion of myocardial cells that have survived. These conditions usually lead to a dilated left ventricle with an increased end-diastolic volume and hence a need to generate greater tension.

EFFECTS OF CARDIAC FAILURE ON OTHER ORGANS

For purposes of description, pathologists usually consider failure of the left and right ventricles as distinct entities. In practice both ventricles function as one unit, and the distinction is less useful from a clinical point of view. Acute processes involving the left ventricle lead to a sudden increase in pulmonary venous pressure and acute pulmonary edema. The best indicator of the degree of pulmonary edema at autopsy is the increase in weight of each lung, often to over 1000g, and the presence of an intra-alveolar exudate on histology. Modern resuscitation techniques often involve the rapid intravenous infusion of fluid, so terminal pulmonary edema is now very common, irrespective of the presence or absence of cardiac failure.

Long-standing elevation of pulmonary venous pressure, classically seen in mitral valve stenosis, leads to a more chronic form of pulmonary edema. Fluid is present in the interalveolar and interlobular septa, and widely-dilated lymphatics are present. Within the alveoli there is a striking feature: macrophages containing hemosiderin, the so-called 'heart failure' cells. In long-standing mitral valve stenosis, the lungs may show mottled shadowing on chest X-ray in life, and at post-mortem they appear brown from the amount of hemosiderin present.

Morphologically, the effects of failure of the right ventricle are best seen in the liver. The cut surface becomes a mottled yellow-red colour, likened to the cut surface of a nutmeg, and centrilobular necrosis is present. While very striking at post-mortem and on histological examination, this form of centrilobular necrosis is neither clinically very important nor pathologically very specific. In life, patients with heart failure do have large livers, but abnormal liver function is rare. The term 'cardiac cirrhosis' is in most instances a complete misnomer.

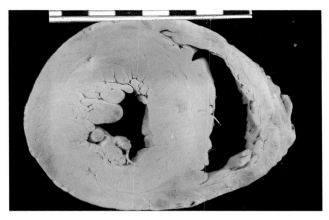

2.1 Left ventricle: pressure overload

2.1 The left ventricle in aortic stenosis: pressure overload. Transverse section of the left and right ventricles in a patient with severe aortic valve stenosis. The left ventricular cavity remains normal in size, but the wall thickness (2.5cm) is markedly increased. The total heart weight was 590g with an isolated left ventricular weight of 280g.

2.2 The left ventricle in aortic valve regurgitation: volume overload. Transverse section of the ventricles in a patient with aortic regurgitation. The total heart weight heart weight was 540g with an isolated left ventricular weight of 290g. As compared with **2.1** the left ventricular cavity is larger but the left ventricular wall thickness is less.

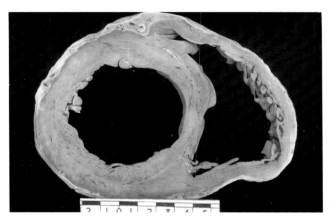

2.2 Left ventricle: volume overload

2.3 Fulton technique for estimation of isolated ventricular mass. In this technique the left ventricle is regarded as a circle of muscle to which the right ventricle is attached. Thus the interventricular septum is part of the left ventricle. The pericardial fat is removed before separating the ventricles for weighing. The technique takes about six minutes per heart and is more easily carried out on a fixed specimen.

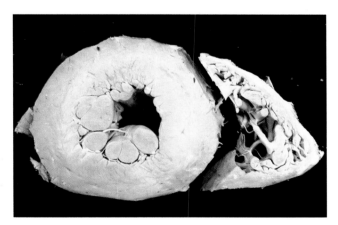

2.3 Fulton technique

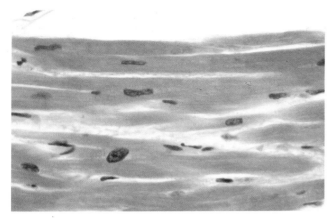

2.4 Normal myocardium

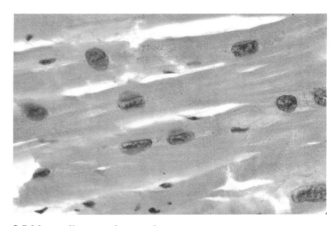

2.5 Myocardium: aortic stenosis

2.4, 2.5 Myocardium in a normal heart and in aortic stenosis. Comparison at same magnification of normal and hypertrophied myocardium due to aortic valve stenosis. In aortic stenosis the muscle fibres are broader and their nuclei larger and more hyperchromatic. These enlarged nuclei are polyploid up to 32N in extreme cases. It is generally thought that in hypertrophy the number of muscle cells does not increase, although the quantitative techniques used to establish this are so complex that some doubt remains.
x375 Hematoxylin and eosin.

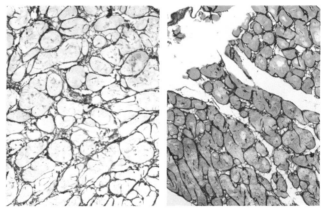

2.6a,b Fibre size in hypertrophy

2.6a, b Measurement of muscle fibre size in hypertrophy. Muscle fibre size is best measured in silver-stained transverse sections. This outlines the muscle cell; a counterstain may or may not be used. Two techniques are employed. In one method the diameter of 100 fibres is measured, but only when a nucleus is present; this is regarded as the maximum diameter of the cell. In the other method all fibres are measured at their short axis, irrespective of whether a nucleus is seen. Subsequently the range and a mean diameter is plotted. In **a** the muscle fibres are increased in diameter although there is considerable scatter in size. This is a case of aortic stenosis. By contrast, in a normal heart **b** the mean fibre diameter is smaller.
x300 Reticulin.

2.7 DNA content of normal and hypertrophied myocardial muscle cells. In a normal adult heart weighing 330g, the majority of cells (53%) are tetraploid. In a hypertrophied heart weighing 600g, the largest single group of cells (43% of the total) are octaploid with an increased number of hexadeploid cells. *(Redrawn from Adler, 1983.)*

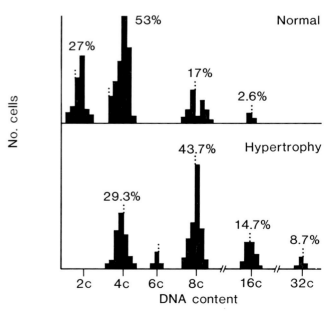

2.7 DNA content of myocardial muscle cells

2.8 Pulmonary edema. Histological section of lung in a patient dying with acute left ventricular failure and pulmonary edema. The alveoli are full of pink-stained protein-rich edema fluid (arrows). The large clear spaces are alveolar ducts which do not flood to the same degree. x25 Hematoxylin and eosin.

2.9 Heart failure cells in the lung. Histological section of lung in a patient with long-standing pulmonary venous hypertension due to mitral valve stenosis. The high pressures in the veins leads to intra alveolar hemorrhage and subsequently the formation, in the alveoli, of macrophages containing iron, the so-called 'heart failure cells'. x225 Hematoxylin and eosin.

2.10 The lung in mitral stenosis. The cut surface of lung showing deep brown pigmentation in long-standing mitral valve stenosis. The specimen is from a museum. Today, the degree of pulmonary venous hypertension needed to produce the change illustrated here would have been treated by valvotomy. The production of this 'brown indurated lung' takes years, and is produced only by mitral valve stenosis in which the patients live for such periods since their left ventricular function is good. Other causes of elevated pulmonary venous pressure are usually associated with left ventricular damage and do not allow sufficient length of survival to develop a brown lung.

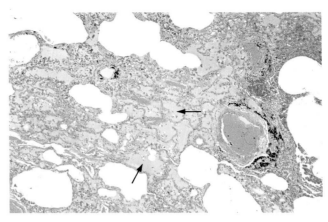
2.8 Pulmonary edema

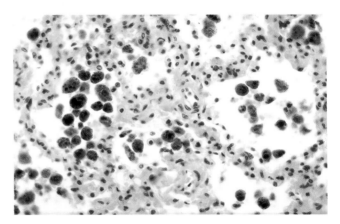
2.9 Heart failure cells

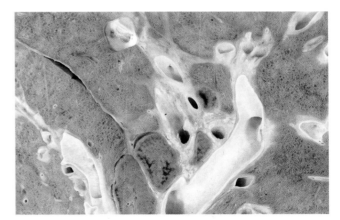
2.10 Lung: mitral stenosis

2.11 The 'nutmeg' liver in cardiac failure. The cut surface of liver from a patient with right heart failure, showing the mottled yellow-red appearance of what is called a 'nutmeg' liver.

2.12 Histological appearances of the liver in right heart failure. Histological sections of a 'nutmeg' liver. In the central zone of the lobules the hepatocytes have vanished, leaving the sinusoids dilated and full of red cells. These are the red areas seen by the naked eye. The more peripheral hepatocytes in the lobule show fatty change. These are the pale areas seen by the naked eye. x25 Hematoxylin and eosin.

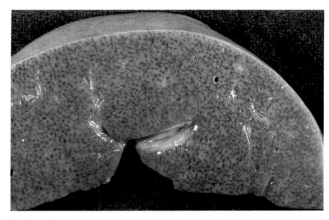

2.11 'Nutmeg' liver

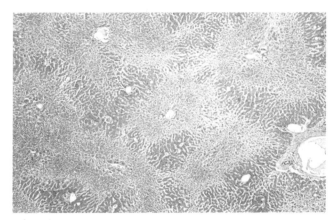

2.12 Liver in right heart failure

CHAPTER 3

Valve Disease

AORTIC STENOSIS
(3.1 – 3.16)

The outflow tract of the left ventricle may be obstructed at one of three levels: valvar, supravalvar and subvalvar. Of these, valve stenosis is by far the most common. Whatever the level of obstruction, the functional effect on the left ventricular myocardium is identical.

Supra-aortic stenosis is an annular constriction in the aorta just above the supra-aortic ridge. The coronary ostia are proximal to the obstruction and tend to enlarge. The disease is familial and may be associated with an abnormal facies.

Stenosis at valvar level arises from several pathological mechanisms. The commonest cause of isolated aortic valve stenosis is dystrophic calcification of a congenital bicuspid valve; the entity is best known as bicuspid calcific aortic valve stenosis. Bicuspid valves occur in around 1% of the normal population at birth. Therefore 1% of the population is at risk of developing aortic valve stenosis by 40 to 50 years of age. Since it is clear that 1% of the population does not develop aortic valve stenosis, there must be considerable variation in the susceptibility of individuals to develop cusp calcification, the causes of which are unknown. Uncalcified bicuspid valves are found coincidentally in post-mortem examinations performed on elderly subjects. Where calcification occurs, it is dystrophic in type, developing within the fibrosa of the valve and projecting outward onto the aortic aspect. The calcific mass may undergo ulceration with development of superimposed surface thrombosis. The calcification found in bicuspid valves is not apparently different from that which develops at a much later age in tricuspid aortic valves. When such calcification in a tricuspid aortic valve produces obstruction to left ventricular outflow, it is best known as 'senile' or tricuspid calcific aortic valve stenosis. The entity is rare under the age of 70 but thereafter becomes more common.

Chronic rheumatic valve disease characteristically produces combinations of aortic stenosis and regurgitation. Chronic rheumatic valve disease is characterized by two pathological processes: fusion of the commissures, i.e. adhesion of cusps together to restrict their opening; and cusp fibrosis. It is the former process which produces valve stenosis. Cusp fibrosis leads to cusp thickening and shortening, and primarily produces valve regurgitation, but it can contribute to valve stenosis, particularly if calcification has developed. Most valves affected by rheumatic disease show combinations of the two basic processes, although pure stenosis or regurgitation can occur. The other hallmark of chronic rheumatic valve disease is that both the aortic and mitral valves are involved.

While the majority of cases of acquired aortic valve stenosis can be fitted into the categories already mentioned, a small minority cannot. The most common unclassifiable form has fusion of one commissure with considerable cusp calcification. Whether this entity is a variant of rheumatic disease is unclear.

The term 'congenital aortic valve stenosis' should be used only when obstruction is present at or soon after birth. It occurs with valves which are essentially a fibrous diaphragm with a central hole. Another variant is the so-called unicommissural valve. True congenital aortic valvar stenosis is the analogue of isolated congenital pulmonary valve stenosis.

Sub-aortic obstruction to the left ventricular outflow may be purely membranous, resulting from a congenital diaphragm that extends from just below the aortic valve to stretch across and become fused to the anterior cusp of the mitral valve. Membranous subaortic stenosis covers the complete range from a simple fibrous diaphragm, which can be easily excised, to a complex tunnel of fibrous tissue which incorporates the anterior cusp of the mitral valve. This malformation as far more difficult to correct surgically.

Purely muscular sub-aortic stenosis occurs when the interventricular septum bulges across beneath the aortic valve to impinge on the anterior cusp of the mitral valve. The enlarged mass of muscle may be the result of septal involvement in hypertrophic cardiomyopathy. In such cases it shows the typical histological appearances of myocardial disarray (Chapter 7). The interventricular septum is, however, normally curved (catenoid) in shape, as seen in a long axis view of the left ventricular outflow, and even in normal compensatory hypertrophy the upper portion may bulge sufficiently to the left to give a degree of outflow obstruction.

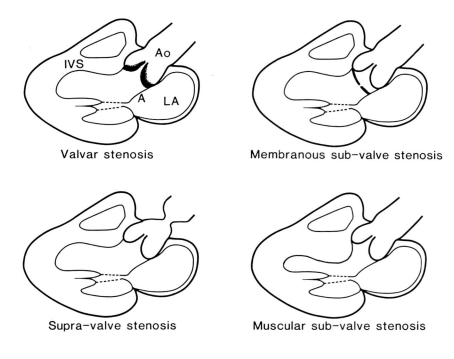

Valvar stenosis

Membranous sub-valve stenosis

Supra-valve stenosis

Muscular sub-valve stenosis

3.1 Left ventricular outflow obstruction

3.1 Left ventricular outflow obstruction. The levels at which left ventricular outflow obstruction can occur. The diagrams represent a long-axis echocardiographic plane and highlight the fact that the anterior cusp of the mitral valve (A) is one component of the left ventricular outflow at sub valve level. The other component is the interventricular septum (IVS). Obstruction can occur above the valve, at the valve or below the valve. Below the valve, obstruction arises either from muscular hypertrophy of the interventricular septum, or from a membrane.

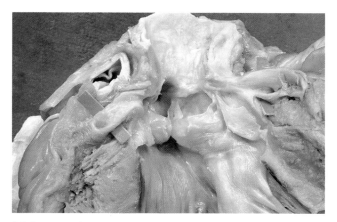

3.2 Supra-aortic stenosis

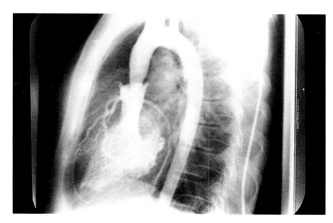

3.3 Supra-aortic stenosis: angiography

3.2 Supra-aortic stenosis. Supra-aortic stenosis in a woman dying suddenly at a young age. There is an annular constriction of the ascending aorta just above the supra-aortic ridge. The coronary arteries are enlarged (red markers).

3.3 Supra-aortic stenosis – angiography. Supra-aortic stenosis demonstrated by angiography. The coronary arteries are dilated and just above their orifices the aorta is drawn in as a 'waist-like' narrowing. The condition was also present in a sibling and the mother of this case.

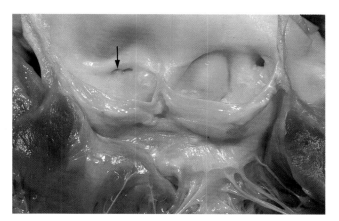

3.4 Bicuspid aortic valve

3.4 Bicuspid aortic valve. Bicuspid aortic valve which was a coincidental finding at post-mortem in a patient with carcinoma. The two cusps are individually normal. One coronary artery opens from each sinus of Valsalva. The right sinus has the conus branch (arrow) to the outflow tract of the right ventricle opening by a separate orifice.

3.5 Bicuspid aortic valve. Bicuspid aortic valve also as a coincidental finding at post-mortem. In this case one cusp is very abnormal: it is large with a thick raphe across the centre which bisects the sinus. One coronary artery arises from each side of the raphe.

This form of bicuspid aortic valve creates some semantic difficulty. It is regarded by some as an acquired fusion of one commissure of a tricuspid aortic valve in the fetal or neonatal stage. All transitions are found, however, between the valves shown in **3.4** and **3.5**; these represent the extremes of a continous spectrum.

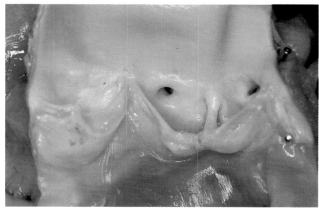

3.5 Bicuspid aortic valve

3.6 Bicuspid calcific aortic valve stenosis. Bicuspid calcific aortic valve stenosis viewed from the aorta with the valve ring intact. There are two cusps both replaced by nodular masses of calcium and there is a slit-like transverse valve orifice. A residual raphe can be seen in the larger cusp. The general view now held is that patients with aortic valve stenosis are not protected from coronary atheroma. Angina in these patients may, therefore, be due either to left ventricular hypertrophy or to coronary stenosis. It may also be due to a combination of both these conditions.

3.7 Bicuspid calcific aortic valve stenosis. Bicuspid calcific aortic valve stenosis viewed from the aortic aspect. The valve orifice is a transverse slit. There is concave defect in the free edge of the larger cusp related to a raphe. This larger cusp is held out across the outflow tract by the rigidity of the raphe. What cusp movement that is retained is in the smaller non-strutted cusp. The commissures are not fused.

3.8 Bicuspid calcific aortic valve stenosis. Bicuspid calcific aortic valve stenosis – the same valve as **3.7** viewed from the ventricular surface. From this aspect the fact that there are two cusps and a transverse opening is more easily apparent.

References:

Davies M J. Pathology of Cardiac Valves. London: Butterworths 1980.

Exadactylos N, Sugrue D D and Oakley C M. Prevalence of coronary artery disease in patients with isolated aortic valve stenosis. Br Heart J 1984; 51: 121-124.

Pomerance A. The pathogenesis of aortic stenosis and its relation to age. Br Heart J 1972; 34: 569-574.

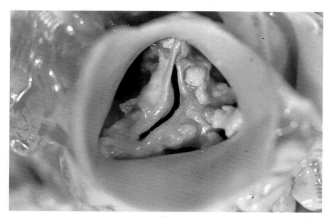

3.6 Bicuspid calcific aortic valve stenosis

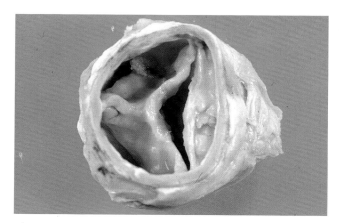

3.7 Bicuspid calcific aortic valve stenosis

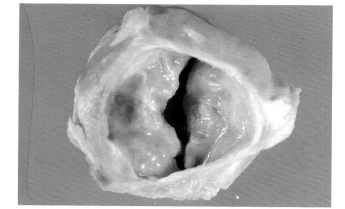

3.8 Bicuspid calcific aortic valve stenosis

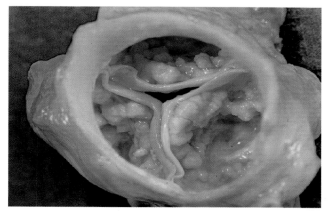

3.9 Tricuspid calcific aortic valve stenosis

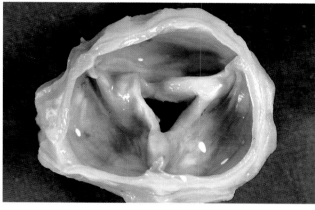

3.11 Rheumatic aortic stenosis

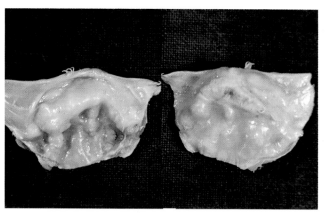

3.10 Age-related aortic calcification

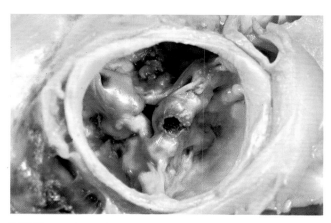

3.12 Rheumatic aortic stenosis

3.9 Tricuspid calcific aortic valve stenosis. Tricuspid calcific aortic valve stenosis of the senile type viewed from the aorta with the ring kept intact. There are three cusps without commissural fusion, and each contains nodular masses of calcium. The cusps, however, meet and the valve was not regurgitant, although it was very difficult to force open and caused significant obstruction to outflow in life.

3.10 Age-related aortic cusp calcification. One valve cusp from **3.9** excised and viewed from the aortic and then from the ventricular surface. The calcification is seen to be a C-shaped mass in the area of maximum cusp flexion. The calcium projects more toward the aortic aspect.

3.11 Rheumatic aortic valve stenosis. Rheumatic aortic valve stenosis in a young patient. The valve is tricuspid, with symmetrical fusion of all three commissures. The result is a central triangular orifice which remained the same size in systole and diastole and produced a mixture of stenosis and regurgitation.

3.12 Rheumatic aortic valve stenosis. Rheumatic aortic valve stenosis in a patient over 60 years of age. Superimposed on the symmetrical commissural fusion there are now large masses of dystrophic calcification in the cusps. Some of these masses have ulcerated onto the aortic surface of the cusp. The development of calcification is characteristic of the older patient with chronic rheumatic valve disease.

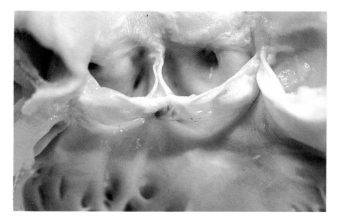

3.13 Idiopathic commissural fusion

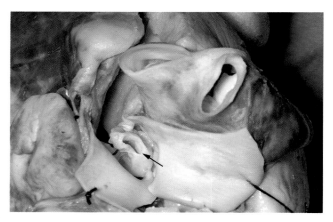

3.14 Congenital aortic stenosis

3.13 Idiopathic aortic commissural fusion. Commissural fusion between two adjacent hemicusps viewed in an opened aortic valve. True commissural fusion, as is the case here, can usually be distinguished from a raphe by the fact that the free edges of the two cusps can be traced into, and recognized in, the fused area. Rheumatic commissural fusion is usually but not inevitably symmetrical, affecting all the commissures. The form of isolated commissural fusion shown here produces an appearance very like a true congenital bicuspid valve, and calcification late in life may produce stenosis. The etiology is unknown. The condition is clumsily called an acquired pseudo-congenital bicuspid valve.

3.14 Congenital aortic stenosis at valve level. Aortic valve stenosis in an infant. The valve is a convex cone of fibrous tissue with a central hole (arrow) and no recognizable free cusps. Many cases of congenital aortic valve stenosis are fatal unless treated early in childhood.

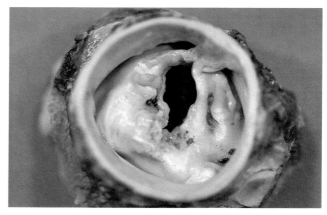

3.15 Unicommissural aortic stenosis

3.15 Unicommissural congenital aortic valve stenosis. Aortic valve stenosis due to a congenital unicommissural valve viewed from above. The aperture is an oval and eccentric hole in fibrous diaphragm which has undergone some calcification. Some cases of unicommissural valves, even when not surgically treated, reach the second or third decade before causing death.

3.16 Membranous subaortic valve stenosis. Membranous subaortic valve stenosis with the left ventricular outflow tract opened through the aortic valve. A fibrous ridge (arrow) runs across the muscular septum just below the aortic valve and fuses into the anterior cusp (A) of the mitral valve.

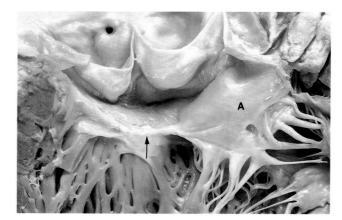

3.16 Membranous subaortic stenosis

AORTIC REGURGITATION
(3.17 – 3.50)

When tested under hemodynamic pressure in the post-mortem room, the normal aortic valve is extremely efficient, closing tightly. Inspection of such a closed valve from the aortic aspect shows that to maintain competence:

(1) the cusps must be intact;

(2) they must exceed in total area the root of the aorta, with the corollary that the cusps must not be reduced in size or the root enlarged;

(3) they are firmly and symmetrically attached to the aortic root at the commissures;

(4) the cusps support each other in the closed position and do not collapse (prolapse) into the ventricle. This support is dependent both on the inherent semilunar shape of the valve cusps, and on their mutual support of each other by the abutting of their ventricular surfaces.

These basic requirements for competence provide a simple scheme for the classification of the causes of incompetence.

At cusp level, perforation of valve cusps through the central portion is characteristic of treated bacterial endocarditis. The perforation is consequent upon the necrosis of connective tissue that occurs beneath the vegetations in the acute phase.

Marked reduction in cusp area with the formation of small rigid cusps is characteristic of chronic rheumatic disease. There can also be spontaneous and traumatic tears of an apparently normal cusp from the root; the antecedents of the former are likely to be inherited weakness of connective tissues, including Marfan's disease. Patients with bicuspid aortic valves usually develop stenosis (see above) but a small proportion develop pure regurgitation in middle life. This occurs in two situations: first, with valves in which there is a marked disproportion in cusp size; and second, in association with aortic root dilatation. There appears to be an undue association of bicuspid valves with idiopathic aortic root dilatation.

The second major subgroup of conditions causing aortic regurgitation are diseases of the aortic root rather than the cusps. The size of the aortic root is dependent on the normal structure of the aortic media just above the supra-aortic ridge. Two disease processes occur at this site, inflammatory aortitis and a non-inflammatory degeneration or 'aortopathy'. The former both dilates and distorts the aortic root, the latter leads to pure dilation.

The term 'aortitis' implies the presence of chronic inflammatory cells of all types within the destroyed elastic tissue of the media. Such a histological picture occurs in syphilis, ankylosing spondylitis and other HLAB27 related diseases, Reiter's syndrome and psoriatic aortitis. There are some morphological features which will distinguish these cases but usually the pathologist is heavily dependent on the serology and other clinical data. In ankylosing spondylitis the aortitis may precede joint symptoms. An aortitis without apparent clinical cause is best referred to as 'non-specific aortitis'. One type is characterized by the formation of numerous giant cells alongside plates of necrotic elastic tissue. This form, known as giant cell aortitis, may be associated with temporal arteritis and polymyalgia rheumatica. The patients have a high ESR and the disease may progress to culminate in an aortic aneurysm and rupture.

In the United Kingdom, there is an increasing number of patients whose aortic root has become dilated but shows no inflammatory element in the media on microscopy. The root diameter is greater than the normal figure of 3.5cm. The intima of the ascending aorta may be wrinkled as in aortitis, but the aortic wall is thinner. Microscopically, varying degrees of destruction of the media are found without any inflammatory cells. The destruction can take the form of focal round areas, or of the inner half of the media, or it may be virtually complete. Cystic areas with acid mucopolysaccharide accumulation may or may not be present. The appearances are variable and while the term cystic medial necrosis is used, this is often strictly a misnomer. Some of these patients are known to have other stigmata of a systemic connective tissue disorder, such as Marfan's disease, osteogenesis imperfecta, or Ehlers-Danlos syndrome. The majority do not, however, and the condition is best known as idiopathic aortic root dilatation. Whether this is a 'forme fruste' of Marfan's disease is as yet uncertain, but some cases are familial. At present, the whole terminology of non-inflammatory aortic medial disease is confused and chaotic, both at a clinical and at a morphological level.

The support and attachment of the cusps to the aortic root is also important in maintaining competence. Dissection tears in the aorta, just above the valve, allow a flap of intima and a cusp to prolapse downward, producing acute aortic regurgitation. Those rare patients who survive are left with permanent regurgitation.

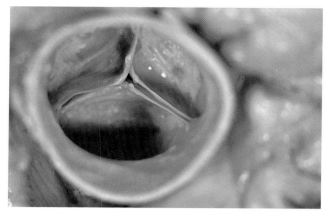

3.17 Closed aortic valve

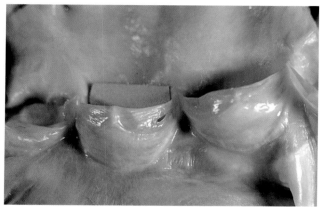

3.18 Normal valve cusps

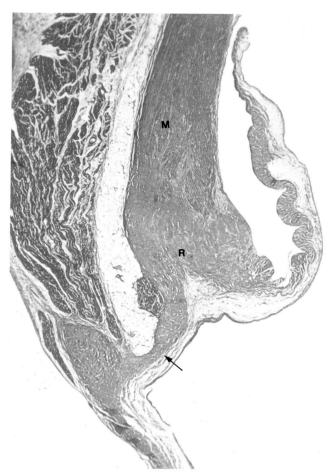

3.19 Normal aortic root: histology

3.17 Normal aortic valve in the closed position.
Normal aortic valve fixed in the closed position at hydro-static pressure equivalent to 100mm Hg. The three cusps meet at the commissures which are attached to the supra-aortic ridge. This ridge marks where the aorta is fused onto the fibrous sleeve or ring of the aortic valve. The fibrous sleeve which contains the cusps bulges outwards under pressure, as the sinus of Valsalva. The cusps abut onto each other over a portion of their ventricular surface.

3.18 Normal aortic valve cusps. Opened aortic valve to give an 'en face' view of the cusps. Each cusp has a central nodule on the free edge from which a line curves downward on each side. This is the closure line above

which the cusp tissue is only supportive and often contains small perforations which are entirely normal. Below the closure line, the body of the cusp actually separates aorta and ventricle when the valve is closed.

3.19 Histological structure of the normal aortic root. Longitudinal histological section through an aortic valve cusp. The collagen of the valve ring (light blue) (R) interdigiatates with the purple-stained muscle of the aortic media (M). The collagen of the valve ring continues into the cusp itself on the aortic aspect. Note that the aortic valve ring is attached (arrow) to the collagen of the anterior cusp of the mitral valve.
x18 Picro-Mallory trichrome.

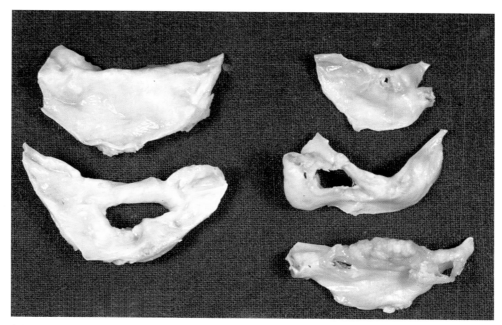

3.20 Aortic regurgitation: bacterial endocarditis

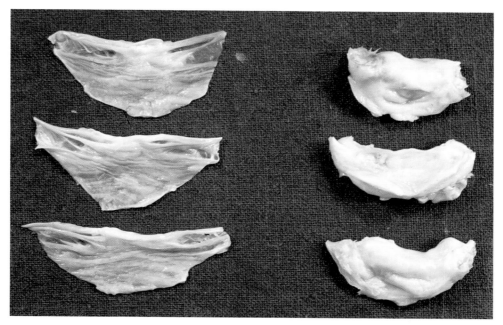

3.21 Aortic cusps in regurgitation

3.20 Aortic regurgitation due to bacterial endocarditis. Aortic valves excised surgically for control of aortic regurgitation following bacterial endocarditis. One valve was bicuspid and the other tricuspid. Both valves show resolving vegetations with perforations of the cusps.

3.21 Comparison of the aortic cusps in regurgitation due to cusp and root disease. Surgically-excised aortic valve cusps are shown, on the left, from a patient with aortic regurgitation due to root dilatation. The cusps are normal in size and thin, almost translucent. Only along the free edge is there a slight linear thickening which occurs as a result of regurgitant flow across the valve. On the right, from a patient with rheumatic aortic regurgitation, there is a marked reduction in the cusp area and an increase in thickness of the cusps.

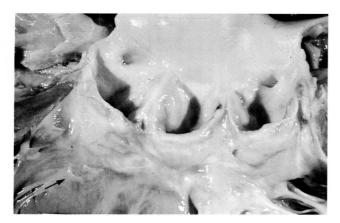

3.22 Rheumatic aortic regurgitation

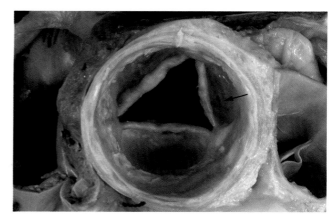

3.23 Syphilitic aortic regurgitation

3.22   Rheumatic aortic regurgitation. Opened aortic valve in a patient with aortic regurgitation of rheumatic type. One commissure shows minimal fusion, and all three cusps are thickened and shortened. On the interventricular septum below the valve are two small semicircular areas of endocardial thickening (arrow), jet lesions, which represent fibrosis where a regurgitant stream has flowed back across the closed valve, hitting the septum.

3.23   Syphilitic aortic regurgitation. The aortic valve has been fixed in the closed position and is seen from the aorta. The cusps fail to meet over a large central area due to dilation of the aortic root and a widening of the commissures (arrow). This widening means the cusp attachments are separated. Each cusp has marked nodular thickening over the free edge as a secondary result of regurgitant flow.

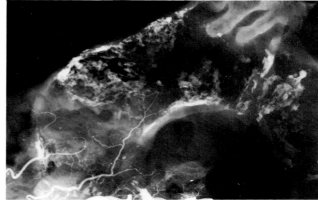

3.23a Syphilitic aortitis: X ray

3.23a   Syphilitic aortitis – X ray. In syphilitic aortitis the whole ascending aorta develops a mottled appearance due to calcification.

3.24   Aortic valve involvement in rheumatoid arthritis. Rheumatoid arthritis involving the aortic and mitral valves. The right and non-coronary cusps of the aortic valve are fused at the commissure and show fibrous thickening of the base of the cusp which extends into the base of the mitral valve (arrow). Aortic regurgitation resulted from the distortion of the root. Extension of the granulomatous process into the body of a cusp is typical of rheumatoid disease.

3.25   Aortic valve involvement in rheumatoid arthritis. Rheumatoid granulomata at the base of an aortic cusp. The endocardial elastic tissue is thickened and eosinophilic. Superficial to this layer, the endocardium is thickened by a mixture of smooth muscle and fibroblastic cells. This feature is seen in both ankylosing spondylitis and rheumatoid disease. The specific feature of rheumatoid disease is the amorphous eosinophilic band of necrosis beneath the endocardium, at the margins of which are histiocytic and chronic inflammatory cells.
x60 Hematoxylin and eosin.

Reference:

Ansell B M and Simkin P A eds. The Heart and Rheumatic Disease. London: Butterworths 1984.

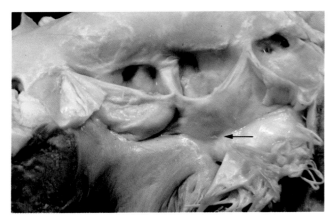

3.24 Aortic valve: rheumatoid arthritis

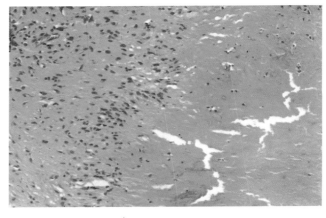

3.26 Rheumatoid granuloma

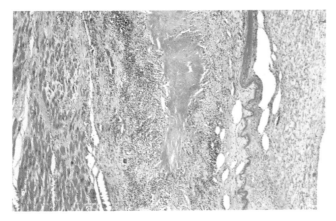

3.25 Aortic valve: rheumatoid arthritis

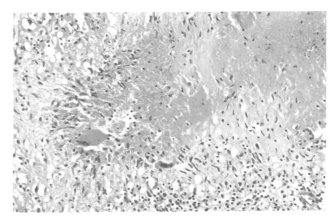

3.27 Rheumatoid granuloma

3.26 Rheumatoid granuloma. The typical palisaded histiocytes at the margins of the area of necrosis in a rheumatoid nodule in the base of an aortic cusp.
x150 Hematoxylin and eosin.

3.27 Rheumatoid granuloma. Rheumatoid involvement of the heart in which the granulomata have an intensely eosinophilic central zone of necrosis with the formation of small giant cells as well as histiocytes. The appearances at histological level are not easy to distinguish from syphilis, although the clinical history and macroscopic appearances usually distinguish the two conditions.
x175 Hematoxylin and eosin.

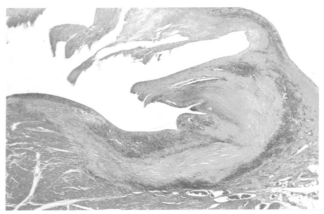

3.28 Rheumatoid granuloma

3.28 Rheumatoid granuloma: mitral valve. Rheumatoid involvement of the mitral valve. A granuloma with a central zone of fibrinoid necrosis and a peripheral band of histiocytes and lymphocytes is present in the angle between the posterior cusp of the mitral valve and the ventricular wall. This is a very common site and is worth a routine section even when the heart looks otherwise normal in a patient with rheumatoid arthritis.
x12 Hematoxylin and eosin.

3.29 Aortic regurgitation due to ankylosing spondylitis. Aortic regurgitation due to aortitis related to ankylosing spondylitis. The intimal surface of the first centimetre of the aorta and the sinuses of Valsava is thick and white, leading to some distortion of the commissures and cusps. The superficial coat of fibrous tissue extends down onto the membranous interventricular septum below the aortic valve and it also involves the base of the anterior cusp of the mitral valve. This extension below the valve is typical of the aortitis associated with the HLAB27 antigen.

3.30 Aortic regurgitation due to ankylosing spondylitis. Histological section across the central fibrous body in ankylosing spondylitis. The connective tissue of the central fibrous body has extended out into the atrial muscle destroying the atrioventricular node, the site of which can be recognized only by the nodal artery (arrow). The expanding connective tissue contains numerous lymphocytes and plasma cells. Its extension from the aortic root into the node, which is anatomically very close, means that around 15% of patients with aortic regurgitation in ankylosing spondylitis develop heart block with a risk of sudden death.
x25 Hematoxylin and eosin.

3.31 Ankylosing spondylitis: small vessel change. Higher-power view of part of **3.30.** The nodal artery shows intimal proliferation and perivascular adventitial fibrosis containing lymphocytes and plasma cells. These vascular changes are highly characteristic of involvement of the heart in ankylosing spondylitis.
x95 Hematoxylin and eosin.

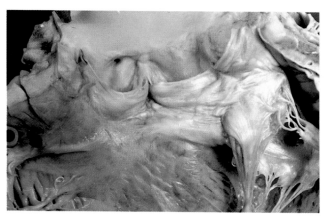

3.29 Aortic regurgitation: ankylosing spondylitis

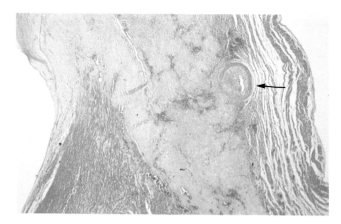

3.30 Aortic regurgitation: ankylosing spondylitis

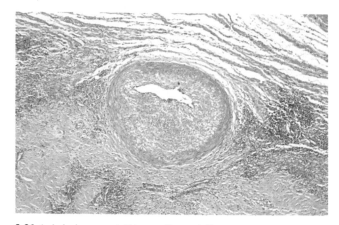

3.31 Ankylosing spondylitis: small vessel disease

References:

Bulkley B H and Roberts W C. Ankylosing spondylitis and aortic regurgitation – description of the characteristic cardiovascular lesion from study of eight necropsy patients. Circulation 1973; 48: 1014-1027.

Bulkley B H and Roberts W C. The heart in systemic lupus erythematosus and the changes induced in it by cortico steroid therapy – a study of 36 necropsy patients. Am J Med 1975; 58: 243-264.

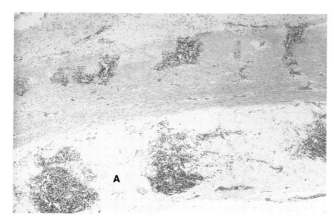

3.32 Syphilitic aortitis

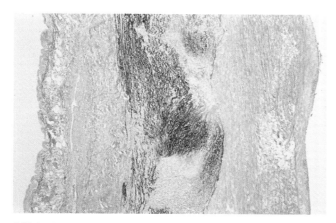

3.33 Syphilitic aortitis

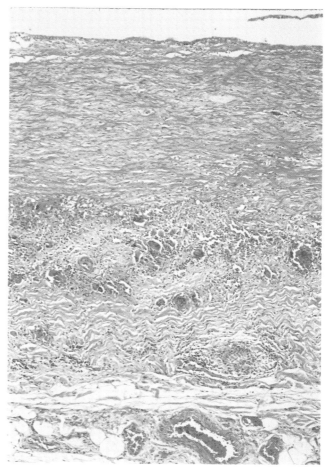

3.34 Syphilitic aortitis

3.32 Syphilitic aortitis. The adventitia (A) is markedly thickened and contains focal collections of lymphocytes and plasma cells. The media also contains similar focal packets of chronic inflammatory cells particularly around the vasa vasorum.
x25 Hematoxylin and eosin.

3.33 Syphilitic aortitis: late stage. The adventitia and intima are thickened, the media thinned. The media has focal areas in which the elastic laminae are totally de-stroyed. These areas are often round. According to the literature, they are related to vasa vasorum but can seldom be actually recognized as such at this late stage.
x25 Elastic-van Gieson.

3.34 Syphilitic aortitis: acute stage. In the acute form the adventitia is markedly thickened and contains numerous giant cell granulatoma with some central necrosis which are beginning to extend into the media.
x40 Hematoxylin and eosin.

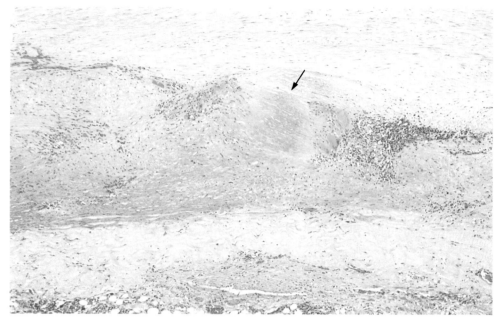

3.35 Giant-cell aortitis

3.35 Giant-cell aortitis. Histological section of the aortic media in a case of giant-cell aortitis. There are acellular necrotic zones (arrow) within the media in which the elastic laminae are still recognizable as refractile strands. There is also a heavy chronic inflammatory cell infiltration in the media.
x40 Hematoxylin and eosin.

3.36 Giant-cell aortitis. Histological section of the aortic media in a case of giant-cell aortitis. At the margins of the necrotic material are chronic inflammatory cells and giants in relation to the areas of the necrotic elastic.
x150 Hematoxylin and eosin.

3.37 Giant-cell aortitis. The intimal surface of the descending aorta in giant-cell aortitis. The intima is wrinkled with longitudinal furrows as well as more 'cobbled' areas and 'pearly' plaques around the intercostal artery orifices. These appearances merely indicate destruction of the underlying media rather than any specific etiology. They are not specific for syphilis or even inflammatory media destruction.

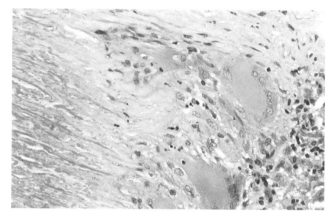

3.36 Giant-cell aortitis

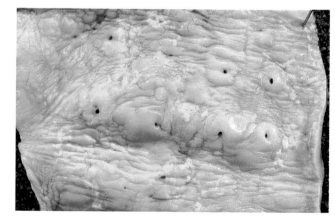

3.37 Giant-cell aortitis

3.38 Aortic regurgitatation due to aortic root dilatation. The valve has been opened in the conventional manner. The circumference of the aortic root at the level of the valve commissures was 11cm. There is a 'jet' lesion on the ventricular septum. The intima of the ascending aorta is thickened with quite extensive lipid deposition and pearly-white plaques. This 'accelerated' atheroma is typical of underlying medial damage and occurs in inflammatory aortitis as well as in non-inflammatory medial degeneration.

3.39 Aortic regurgitation due to non-inflammatory aortic root dilatation. The valve has been fixed in the closed position and the ring kept intact. It may thus be clearly seen whether the valve is competent. The ring is dilated with a diameter of 4.3cm. The valve cusps do not meet to close the valve aperture in the central area. The right coronary cusp has slipped under the left coronary cusp, 'prolapsing' down into the ventricle. This follows the reduction in overlap of the cusps as the root dilates. The cusp has a very distinct fibrous rolled edge but the body of the cusp is normal. This fibrosis is the secondary effect of regurgitant flow over the cusp edge and should not be confused with rheumatic fibrosis which involves the cusp body.

3.40 Aortic regurgitation: secondary cusp changes. Histological section across the right coronary aortic valve cusp shown in **3.39**. The free edge of the cusp is replaced by a round nodule of collagenous tissue but the cusp body is of normal width.
x20 Van Gieson.

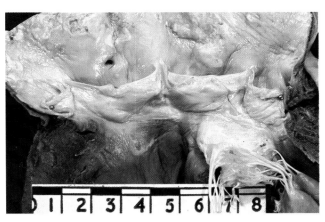
3.39 Aortic regurgitation: root dilatation

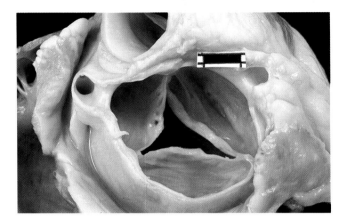
3.38 Aortic regurgitation: root dilatation

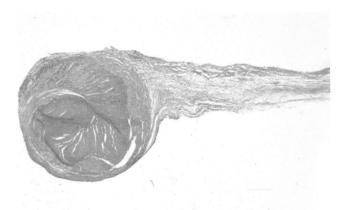
3.40 Aortic regurgitation: cusp changes

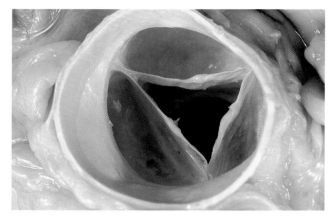

3.41 Aortic regurgitation: root dilation

3.43 Aortic media: root dilation

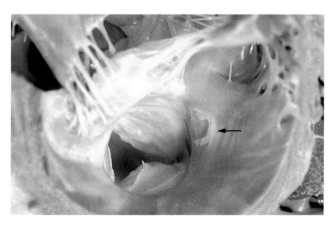

3.42 Jet lesion: aortic regurgitation

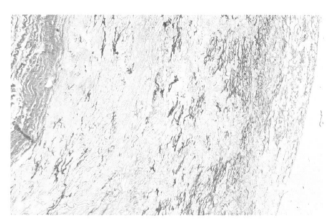

3.44 Aortic media: root dilation

3.41 Aortic regurgitation due to non-inflammatory root dilation. The valve has been fixed in the closed position and viewed from the aorta. The cusps fail to meet over a large area in the centre but none have prolapsed downward and there is no thickening of the cusp edges, suggesting that the regurgitant jet was over a wide central area. Aortic root dilation is a typical finding in Marfan's disease.

3.42 Jet lesion in aortic regurgitation. The same valve as in **3.41** viewed from below, looking up through the aortic valve from the ventricle. The central area where the cusps fail to meet is opposite a well-marked semilunar endocardial jet lesion (arrow) on the ventricular septum.

3.43, 3.44 Aortic media in non-inflammatory root disease. The aortic media just above the aortic root (**3.43**) in a normal heart, and (**3.44**) in aortic regurgitation due to non-inflammatory root dilatation. The normal media (**3.43**) has regularly-arranged elastic laminae throughout its width. The abnormal media (**3.44**) has lost many of the laminae in the outer two-thirds. In this zone only a few irregular fragments of elastic remain. The elastic tissue has been replaced by loose connective tissue but there are no cystic spaces.
x35 Elastic-van Gieson.

Reference:

Roberts W C and Honig H S. The spectrum of cardiovascular disease in the Marfan Syndrome. A clinico-morphologic study of 18 necropsy patients and comparison to 151 previously reported necropsy patients. Am Heart J 1982; 104: 115-135.

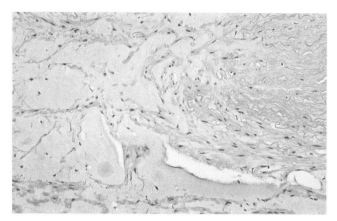

3.45 Aortic media: root dilation

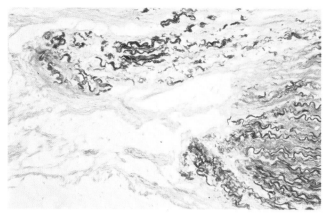

3.46 Aortic media: root dilation

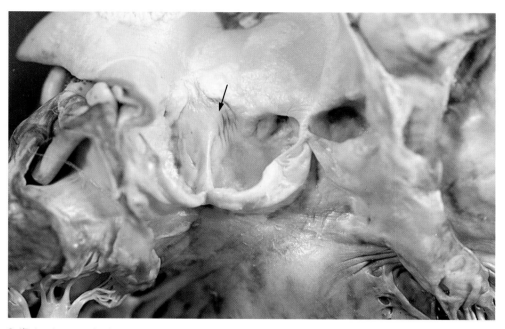

3.47 Aortic regurgitation: healed dissection tear

3.45 Aortic media in non-inflammatory root dilation. The media contains cystic spaces containing blue-staining mucoid material. This change is often known as cystic medial necrosis, but true necrosis is usually absent. ×125 Hematoxylin and eosin.

3.46 Aortic media in non-inflammatory root dilation. The elastic laminae are fragmented and shortened, being very abnormal rather than just pushed aside by the pools of mucin.
×125 Elastic-van Gieson.

3.47 Aortic regurgitation following healed dissection tear. Above one commissure of the valve there is a healed intimal dissection tear (arrow). The commissure has prolapsed down, carrying two cusps with it. The tear has healed leaving the cusp permanently fixed at a lower level.

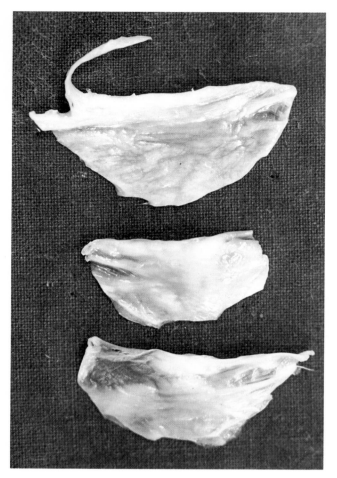

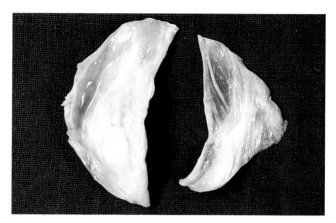

3.49 Bicuspid valve with regurgitation

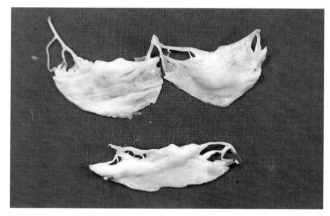

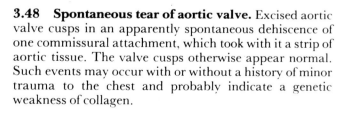

3.48 Spontaneous tear of aortic valve

3.50 Floppy aortic valve

3.48 Spontaneous tear of aortic valve. Excised aortic valve cusps in an apparently spontaneous dehiscence of one commissural attachment, which took with it a strip of aortic tissue. The valve cusps otherwise appear normal. Such events may occur with or without a history of minor trauma to the chest and probably indicate a genetic weakness of collagen.

3.49 Bicuspid aortic valve with regurgitation. Bicuspid aortic valve excised surgically for pure aortic regurgitation. One cusp is larger than the other. Such cusps fail to support each other when closed and one slips under the other.

3.50 Floppy aortic valve cusps. Excised aortic valve cusps in a patient with pure regurgitation and a normal dimension of the root. The valves were soft and gelatinous rather than fibrous and have marked elongation of the lunular areas with excessive fenestration. These changes are regarded as a myxomatous degeneration similar to the floppy mitral valve, but are very much rarer.

CHAPTER 4

Mitral, Tricuspid and Pulmonary Valve Disease

MITRAL VALVE DISEASE
(4.1 – 4.22)

For all practical purposes the sole cause of acquired mitral valve stenosis **(4.1-4.6)** is chronic rheumatic disease.

In its simplest form, fusion of the valve commissures produces a fibrous but still mobile diaphragm with a central oval aperture. Since the valve is still mobile, an opening 'snap' is heard clinically. The critical size of the valve orifice for producing severe clinical disease is 1-1.5 sq cm. From a surgical viewpoint, such valves are easily repaired by simply splitting or reopening the commissures, often via the left atrium as a 'closed' procedure, and thus the operation can be carried out without sophisticated cardiac surgery.

In more complex cases, usually found in older patients, cusp rigidity from dense fibrosis and calcification contribute significantly to obstruction. Calcification in the cusps develops both as nodules and as a more diffuse calcification along the closure line. In some cases, dense fibrosis fusing the papillary muscles and chordae into a tunnel introduces an element of sub-valve stenosis. The presence of severe valve calcification necessitates total replacement of the valve at operation.

In mitral valve stenosis, the left atrial size is very variable, for reasons that are poorly understood. The presence of thrombus within the appendage and more rarely in the cavity of the atrium correlates with the presence of atrial fibrillation, which is itself more common in larger atria. The majority of patients with significant mitral stenosis develop pulmonary hypertension and as a result have right ventricular hypertrophy.

Mitral regurgitation **(4.7-4.22)** has a more complex pathogenesis than mitral stenosis. It is best considered as processes affecting the different components of the valve.

Rheumatic valve disease affects both the cusps and chordae, causing dense fibrosis. The chordae significantly shorten, restricting movement and preventing cusp apposition; cusp fibrosis reduces the cusp area particularly in the posterior cusp, producing an immobile fibrous shelf rather than a mobile structure. In infective endocarditis, perforation of the bodies of the cusps, erosion of cusp edges, ruptured chordae and cusp aneurysms are all the sequelae of destruction of the fibrous tissue of the valve.

The condition that is now widely known as the floppy mitral valve is due to a stretching of the connective tissue, leading to an expansion of the cusp area and elongated thin chordae which may spontaneously rupture. The functional effect on the valve is that in ventricular systole the mitral cusps, particularly the posterior, overshoot and prolapse into the atria allowing regurgitation to develop late in systole. The valve is recognized pathologically by its domed or ballooned shape, and histologically the fibrosa of the valve is replaced by cystic areas containing acid mucopolysaccharides. This is why the entity is known as myxomatous or myxoid valve degeneration. The floppy mitral valve is variously regarded: as a persistence of a fetal-type valve structure; as degeneration in a valve which was anatomically abnormal with lack of cusp support; as an age-related degeneration of collagen; and as a partial failure of collagen synthesis. The last concept is supported by an association of the floppy mitral valve with all of the known genetic defects in collagen synthesis, particularly Marfan's disease.

The clinical term mitral valve prolapse indicates an upward movement of one or both cusps into the atria in ventricular systole and is a diagnosis made by echocardiography. Mitral regurgitation may or may not be present. The term is a clinical one and has no single pathological cause. The majority of patients with significant regurgitation and prolapse do have the expansion of the cusp and histological changes described above as the floppy mitral valve, but others have ischemic papillary muscle damage without a cusp abnormality. The exact pathology of the mitral valve in the 5% of normal young individuals who have mitral valve prolapse, found on routine echocardiography but without regurgitation, is very controversial. An unknown proportion of these subjects will develop a floppy valve and regurgitation, but the risk appears small. The majority of patients with chordal rupture are found to have a floppy valve and myxoid change in both cusp and chordae. In ischemic disease, chordal rupture does not occur since the chordae are avascular but the tip of a papillary muscle, to which only one or two chordae are attached, may tear. Other causes of chordal rupture include bacterial endocarditis, trauma and the acute phase of rheumatic fever. Spontaneous rupture of chordae without other valve abnormalities occasionally occurs and is of unknown cause.

Papillary muscle damage is most commonly the result of ischemic heart disease. A complete spectrum of severity occurs; when there is complete rupture of a head of a papillary muscle in an acute myocardial infarction, torrential mitral regurgitation develops suddenly. At the other extreme, simple scarring following infarction may lead to trivial regurgitation in a high proportion of patients who survive a posterior myocardial infarct.

Over the age of 70, calcification begins to develop in the mitral valve ring. This forms a band of calcific nodules which encircle the atrioventricular ring tucked up under the junction of the cusp with the posterior ventricular wall. The calcific masses are often contiguous with similar nodules developing in the aortic valve. In the mitral valve, the ring, as the result of rigidity, loses its normal ability to reduce in size as the ventricle contracts. This results in a mild degree of regurgitation. True dilatation of the mitral valve ring develops in the recognized genetic abnormalities of collagen including Marfan's disease. In what is called functional mitral regurgitation, the left ventricle is dilated but the valve ring size at autopsy is often only marginally raised. This syndrome of mitral regurgitation, which waxes and wanes with the contractile function of the left ventricle, is considered to result from the outward shift of the base of the papillary muscles that occurs with ventricular dilatation.

References:

Bulkley B H and Roberts W C. Dilatation of the mitral annulus. A rare cause of mitral regurgitation. Am J Med 1975; 59: 457-463.

Burch G E, Depasquale N P and Phillips J H. The syndrome of papillary muscle dysfunction. Am Heart J 1968; 75: 399-415.

Burch G E and Giles T D. Angle of traction of the papillary muscles on normal and dilated hearts. A theoretical analysis of its importance in mitral valve dynamics. Am Heart J 1972; 84: 141-144.

Perloff J W and Roberts W C. The mitral apparatus. Functional anatomy of mitral regurgitation. Circulation 1972; 46: 227-239.

Roberts W C and Perloff J K. Mitral Valvar disease – a clinicopathological survey of the conditions causing the mitral valve to function abnormally. Annals of Internal Medicine 1972; 77: 939-975.

4.1 Mitral valve stenosis due to chronic rheumatic disease. Mitral valve stenosis with the valve viewed from the left atrium. The orifice is small and oval, measuring less than 1 sq cm in area. The stenosis is predominantly due to fusion of both commissures, and the valve is not calcified. The atrium is dilated with diffuse white endocardial thickening but no mural thrombus is present, even in the widely dilated atrial appendage (A).

4.2 Mitral valve stenosis in a surgical specimen. Mitral valve stenosis in a surgical specimen taken at mitral valve replacement. The valve orifice is 1 sq cm in area, being restricted both by commissural fusion between the two cusps and by nodular masses of calcification at both commissures and to a lesser extent in the anterior cusp.

4.3 Mitral valve stenosis at sub-valve level. Mitral valve stenosis viewed from the ventricular surface. The cusps are fused directly onto the papillary muscles by dense pillars of fibrous tissue which cover and incorporate the chordae. This mass of fibrosis produces a sub-valve stenosis, since blood normally enters the ventricle between the chordae. The valve orifice is a tiny slit.

4.4-4.5 Mitral valve stenosis due to rheumatic valve disease. Mitral valve stenosis in patients of similar age and clinical disability. In both the valve is seen fixed open from the left atrium. In **4.4** the atrium is small and in **4.5** large and thin-walled. The mitral valve orifices are of equivalent size; in both the aperture is small and oval, due to commissural fusion and some cusp calcification. Neither atrium contains thrombus.

4.6 Right ventricular hypertrophy in mitral valve stenosis. Transverse section across the left and right ventricles equivalent to short axis view in a patient with pure mitral valve stenosis (same case as **4.4**). The left ventricle is small and greatly exceeded in size by a dilated right ventricle which has a thick wall and very enhanced trabecular pattern.

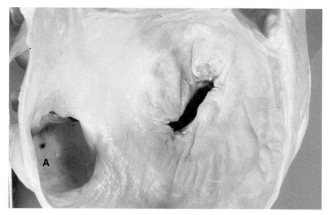

4.1 Chronic rheumatic mitral stenosis

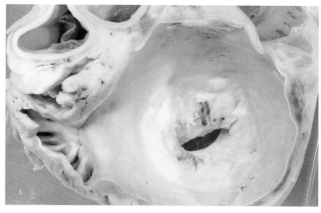

4.4 Rheumatic mitral stenosis

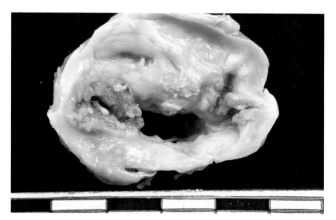

4.2 Mitral stenosis

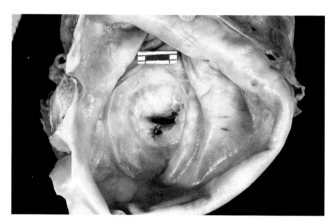

4.5 Rheumatic mitral stenosis

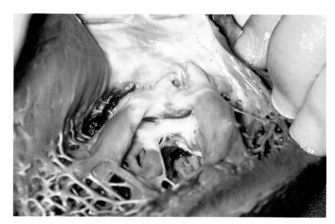

4.3 Mitral valve: sub-valve level

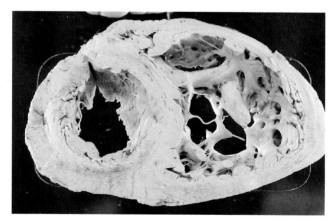

4.6 Mitral stenosis: right ventricular hypertrophy

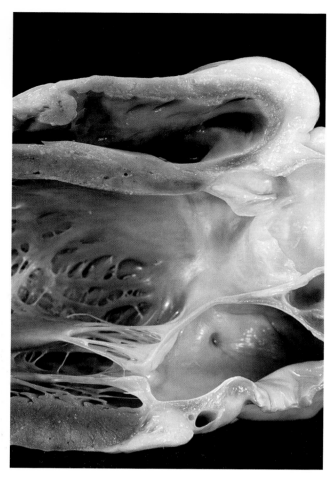

4.7 Normal mitral valve

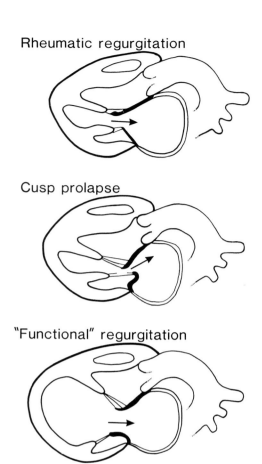

Rheumatic regurgitation

Cusp prolapse

"Functional" regurgitation

4.9 Abnormal mitral valve function

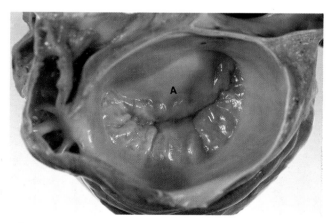

4.8 Normal mitral valve

4.7 Normal mitral valve in the closed position: long axis view. In this long axis view the mitral valve has been closed by hydrostatic pressure in the left ventricle. The essential feature is that the cusps are held in their correct and apposing position by the chordae and papillary muscles which prevent the cusps being blown up into the left atrium (prolapse) during ventricular systole.

4.8 Normal mitral valve in the closed position viewed from the left atrium. The mitral valve is viewed in the closed position from above in the left atrium. The closed valve forms a flat floor to the atrium and neither cusp bulges up into the atrium. The closure line is semilunar pointing anteriorly. The anterior cusp (A) is different in shape from the posterior cusp. The latter is often divided into three 'scallops', medial, central and lateral.

4.9 Diagrammatic representation of abnormal mitral valve function:

A. Rheumatic mitral regurgitation. The chordal shortening attaches the cusps to the apex of the papillary muscles restricting movement. This restriction means that in systole the cusps are unable to meet and a regurgitant jet develops through the central area of the valve.

B. Mitral regurgitation due to prolapse of the posterior cusp. Due to rupture of chordae, in systole a portion of a cusp is blown upwards into the atrium. A regurgitant jet occurs beneath this prolapsed cusp and is often angled to hit the atrial wall close to the aorta. This allows marked transmission of the systolic murmur up into the neck. Any portion of either cusp may prolapse, or in extreme cases both cusps are involved.

C. Functional mitral regurgitation due to left ventricular dilatation. Apposition of the cusps is prevented in a dilated left ventricle by the marked lateral shift of the papillary muscles widening the angle between their long axis.

4.10 Functional mitral regurgitation due to ventricular dilation. Mitral regurgitation due to poor left ventricular contraction in a child with a dilated cardiomyopathy. The mitral ring is not dilated but the ventricle is globular in shape. Severe mitral regurgitation was present in life. There is a nodular thickening (arrow) on the free edge of the anterior cusp – a change which is secondary to longstanding regurgitation. The remainder of the cusp and the chordae are normal.

4.11 Rheumatic mitral regurgitation. Surgically-excised mitral valve in a patient with dominant regurgitation and minimal stenosis due to rheumatic disease. The valve commissures are fused but the actual valve orifice was 2 sq cm in area and not critically stenotic. Calcification extends from the medial commissure into the anterior cusp which was totally immobile and could not move to significantly reduce the size of the valve aperture in ventricular systole.

4.12 Rheumatic mitral regurgitation. Pure mitral regurgitation due to rheumatic disease (surgical specimen). The posterior cusp is a fibrous shelf and reduced in area so that, despite retention of mobility by the anterior cusp, the valve orifice could not close.

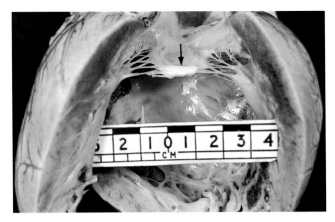

4.10 Functional mitral regurgitation

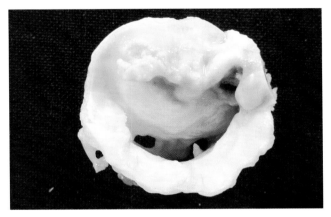

4.11 Rheumatic mitral regurgitation

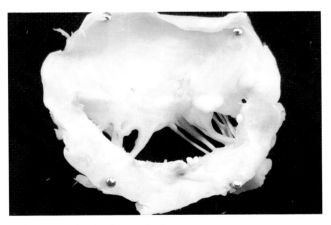

4.12 Rheumatic mitral regurgitation

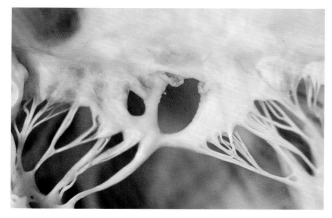

4.13 Mitral regurgitation: bacterial endocarditis

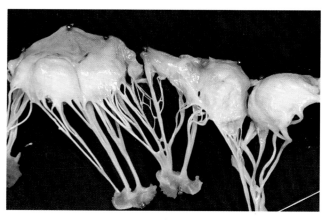

4.15 Floppy mitral valve

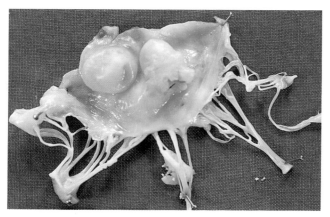

4.14 Mitral regurgitation: bacterial endocarditis

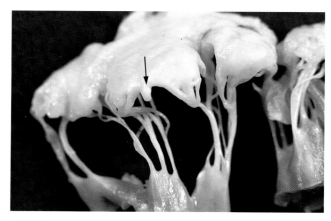

4.16 Floppy mitral valve

4.13 Mitral regurgitation following bacterial endo-carditis. Anterior cusp of the mitral valve in a patient who had severe mitral regurgitation following acute bacterial endocarditis. There are two well-defined smooth-edged holes right through the body of the cusp. A few residual vegetations are present on the edge of the defect. The infecting organism was *Staphylococcus aureus*.

4.14 Mitral regurgitation following bacterial endo-carditis. Anterior cusp of the mitral valve excised at surgery for severe mitral regurgitation following bacterial endocarditis. There are two aneurysmal bulges on the body of the anterior cusp, one of which has ruptured. Infection developed initially on a jet lesion of aortic re-gurgitation on the anterior cusp.

4.15 Floppy mitral valve. Surgically-excised floppy mitral valve. The anterior cusp shows some doming of the free edge but the cusp body is normal. The posterior cusp is dome-shaped and has a thickened, white appearance which affects all three of its scallops. The chordae to both cusps are elongated. The cusps, while becoming white and opaque from surface fibrosis developing secondary to friction and impact due to excessive mobility of the valve, never feel firm and rigid as in rheumatic disease. The most diagnostic feature is the dome shape the cusps adopt.

4.16 Floppy mitral valve. Surgically-excised posterior cusp of a floppy mitral valve. Mitral regurgitation due to cusp prolapse had been present. The scallops of the cusps have the typical dome shape and white opaque surface. There is a stump of a ruptured chorda (arrow).

4.17 Floppy mitral valve. In this case the anterior cusp is minimally affected. The middle scallop of the posterior cusp is domed or ballooned up into the atrium. The chordae of the medial scallop are fused onto the posterior wall of the left ventricle and actually encased in fibrous tissue (arrows). This lesion is the extreme end result of the fibrosis that develops on the endocardium following repeated mechanical trauma due to impact of the chordae in the hypermobile valve.

4.18 Mitral valve prolapse leading to regurgitation in a floppy valve. Function has been simulated in the post-mortem room by placing hydrostatic pressure in the left ventricle and viewing the mitral valve from the atrium. The valve has closed but the dome-shaped middle scallop of the posterior cusp has been pushed up into the atrium and water jets from under its free edge into the atrium.

4.19 Floppy mitral valve – histological appearances. Histological section taken across the posterior cusp of a floppy mitral valve. At the proximal end of the cusp the collagen bundles are densely packed but toward the distal edge the collagen has become much less densely packed, disorganized and with numerous spaces present. These spaces can be shown to contain acid mucopolysaccharides and are the areas of so-called myxoid or myxomatous degeneration.
x18 Elastic-van Gieson.

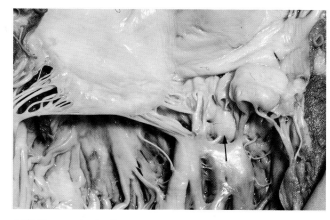

4.17 Floppy mitral valve

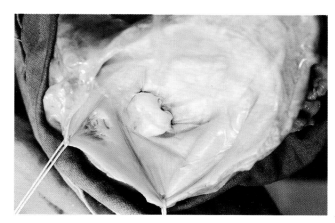

4.18 Floppy mitral valve

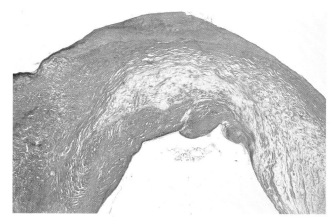

4.19 Floppy mitral valve: histology

References:

Jeresaty R M. Mitral Valve Prolapse. New York: Raven Press 1979.

Pyeritz R E and Wappel M A. Mitral valve dysfunction in the Marfans Syndrome. Clinical and echocardiographic study of prevalence of natural history. Am J Med 1983; 74: 797-807.

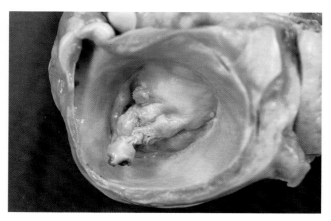

4.20 Papillary muscle rupture

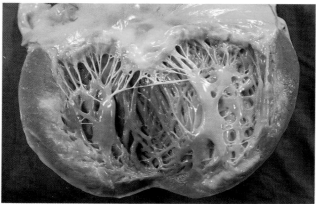

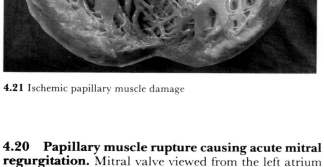

4.21 Ischemic papillary muscle damage

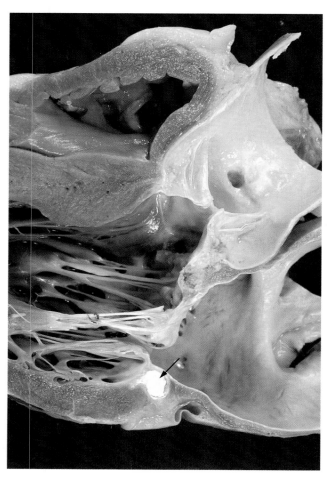

4.22 Mitral ring calcification

4.20 Papillary muscle rupture causing acute mitral regurgitation. Mitral valve viewed from the left atrium in a patient who developed severe regurgitation some days after an acute myocardial infarction. The stump of a ruptured papillary muscle lies in the atrium tangled among chordae. The stump of the papillary muscle continually crosses and recrosses the valve orifice as the cusp flails.

4.21 Mild ischemic papillary muscle damage causing mitral regurgitation. Opened mitral valve in a patient who developed mild mitral regurgitation following a posterior myocardial infarct. As compared to the normal anterolateral papillary muscle, the posterior-medial muscle is paler, thinner and elongated, having been replaced by fibrous tissue. Sub-endocardial scarring is pre-

sent throughout the posterior wall of the left ventricle. Mitral valve prolapse also occurs in this form of ischemic damage.

4.22 Mitral valve: ring calcification. Long axis section across a heart with mitral ring calcification and prolapse of the anterior cusp. There are irregular masses of calcium in the bases of the anterior and posterior cusps. The centre of the calcified material has undergone a liquefying process producing white (sometimes yellow) crumbly material which can be 'washed out' to leave a cavity (arrow). The reason for this change is unknown but it must not be mistaken for tuberculous caseation. The anterior cusp has prolapsed into the atria above the posterior cusp. Ring calcification occurs commonly in old age both with and without previous valve disease.

Reference:

Pomerance A. Pathological and clinical study of calcification of the mitral valve ring. J Clin Pathol 1970; 23: 354-361.

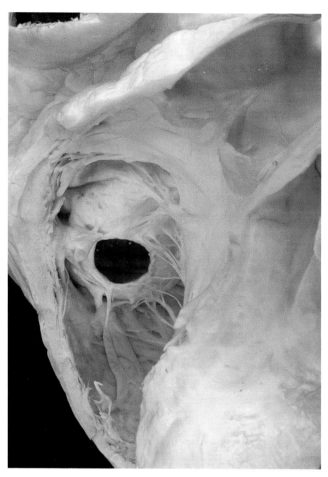

4.23 Rheumatic tricuspid stenosis

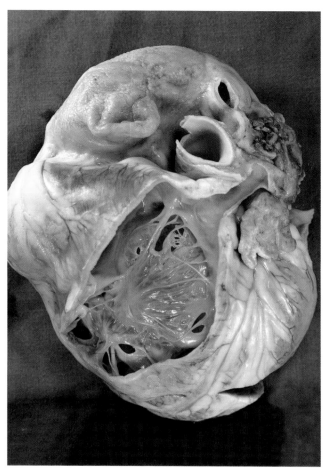

4.24 Ebstein's anomaly

ABNORMALITIES OF THE PULMONARY AND TRICUSPID VALVES (4.23 – 4.28)

Rheumatic disease virtually never involves these valves in isolation, occurring only in association with aortic or mitral disease. Rheumatic tricuspid valve stenosis is due to fusion of the commissures, and it produces a fibrous diaphragm. The dense cusp fibrosis and calcification seen in the mitral valve does not occur.

Ebstein's anomaly of the tricuspid valve is a congenital abnormality in which there is a grossly abnormal valve inserted lower in the ventricle than the atrioventricular ring, thus 'atrializing' a portion of the ventricle. There is a wide spectrum of cusp abnormality, ranging from minimal functional effect to production of tricuspid stenosis caused by the abnormal valve forming a fenestrated sheet hung across the right ventricular outflow.

Solitary ulceration of the tricuspid valve occurs in both acute and chronic pulmonary hypertension. It is a sharply-defined pit in the atrial aspect of the cusp. Repeated healing of such ulcers is probably responsible for the thickening of the tricuspid valve that occurs in long-standing cor pulmonale.

Carcinoid valve disease affects both the pulmonary and tricuspid valves, being recognized as a diffuse sheet of fibrosis covering the leaflets and cusps. The dominant functional effects are incompetence, although as fibrosis develops the pulmonary valve is constricted and pulled in, giving an element of pulmonary stenosis. Most cases occur as a result of metastatic gastro-intestinal carcinoid tumours in the liver. Rare cases of left-sided carcinoid valve disease are recorded with pulmonary tumours.

4.23 Rheumatic tricuspid valve stenosis. The anterior wall of the right ventricle has been removed to display the tricuspid valve from below. The valve is a diaphragm with a central round aperture produced by commissural fusion. The pulmonary valve is not affected by rheumatic disease.

4.24 Ebstein's anomaly. The right ventricle has been opened anteriorly to show the very abnormal tricuspid valve which has been displaced downward, forming a fenestrated curtain across the ventricular cavity.

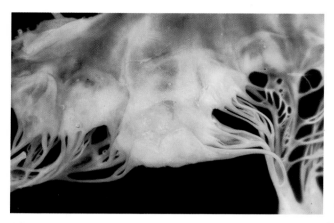

4.25 Tricuspid valve ulceration

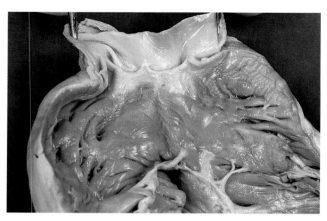

4.27 Pulmonary valve: carcinoid

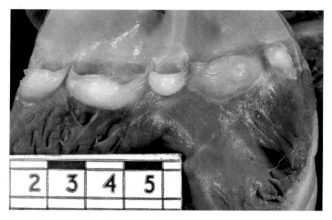

4.26 Pentacuspid pulmonary valve

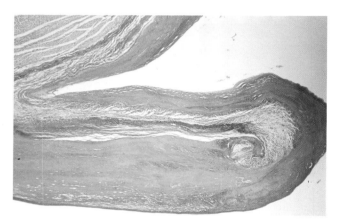

4.28 Pulmonary valve: carcinoid

4.25   Isolated tricuspid valve ulceration. There is an ulcer with a yellow base and hemorrhagic edge in the middle of the anterior cusp. The edge of the cusp appears nodular and thickened, suggesting long-standing pulmonary hypertension. The lesion results from increased impact of the valve cusps when right ventricular pressure is high.

4.26   Pentacuspid pulmonary valve. Bicuspid, quadricuspid and pentacuspid pulmonary valves are not uncommon anatomical variants. They have no pathological sequelae or clinical significance.

4.27   Carcinoid pulmonary valve disease. All three pulmonary cusps are shrunken and fibrotic, with some endocardial thickening which extends on to the ventricular surface of the right ventricular outflow. No macroscopic evidence of thrombus formation is present (cf. endomyocardial fibrosis, Chapter 7).

4.28   Carcinoid pulmonary valve disease: histology. The underlying architecture of the cusp is recognizable by the fine elastic tissue it contains. Both aspects, but particularly the ventricular surface, are covered by a thick layer of red-staining collagen. The fibrous tissue does not contain inflammatory cells. It is thought to represent an ill-understood direct effect of products of the carcinoid tumour such as serotonin on endocardial tissue. x18 Elastic-van Gieson.

Reference:

Pomerance A. Isolated ulceration of the tricuspid valve. J Pathol 1970; 102: 171-177.

CHAPTER 5

Infective Endocarditis

BACTERIAL ENDOCARDITIS
(5.1 – 5.20)

The term infective endocarditis means the direct infection of an endocardial surface, usually that of a valve cusp, from which the organism can be grown. The speed at which the disease progresses and the pattern of complications are to a large extent determined by the characteristics of the infecting micro-organism. The older classification of the disease into acute, sub-acute and chronic merely reflected the time course of the disease and have been largely and correctly superseded by the practice of qualifying the term endocarditis by its organism.

Common to all forms of infective endocarditis is the presence of a mass of thrombus, known as vegetations, on the endocardial surface. These vegetations contain the actively growing organism. Acute rheumatic endocarditis is therefore *not* an example of infective endocarditis. The number of organisms which are known to produce infective endocarditis is large and growing daily as the microbiologist's ability to culture rare and exotic organisms improves. The infecting agent may be bacterial, fungal or rickettsial.

The common bacterial organisms are *Staphylococcus aureus* and streptococci of all groups including both *S.viridans* and *S.fecalis*. *Staphylococcus aureus* produces the archetypal acute bacterial endocarditis with a short course, high fever, no history of a previous valve lesion, rapid evolution of valve regurgitation and septic emboli leading to tissue abscesses from which the organism can be grown. *S.viridans* produces the classic sub-acute bacterial endocarditis with a prolonged course of weeks or months, intermittent low-grade pyrexia, known predisposing cardiac abnormality, slow evolution of valve incompetence, and emboli which lead to bland infarction.

Predisposing Conditions and Pathogenesis

Experimental work suggests that two prerequisites, circulating micro-organisms and small platelet thrombi forming on an endocardial surface, are needed to develop infective endocarditis. The surmised sequence of events is that organisms become incorporated into a mass of platelets. The organism begins to divide, leading to the formation of yet more thrombus. In the enclosed site within a mass of thrombus the organism is relatively protected from phagocytosis by polymorphs, although an acute inflammatory process is rapidly invoked in the underlying valve tissue. Platelet thrombi form on any endocardial surface which is subject to localized high-pressure turbulent blood flow, or where repeated trauma leads to endothelial damage.

In the past, chronic rheumatic valve lesions, particularly those causing aortic and mitral regurgitation, were pre-eminent predisposing causes for bacterial endocarditis. Pure mitral valve stenosis with its low pressure flow has a relatively low risk of becoming infected. With mitral and aortic regurgitation the initial infection may not be on the valve itself but on the patch of fibrous thickening where the regurgitant jet of blood hits the endocardium.

Non-rheumatic causes of mitral regurgitation associated with a risk of bacterial endocarditis include the floppy mitral valve, the cleft mitral anterior cusp in ostium primum atrial septal defects, and hypertrophic cardiomyopathy. Any patient with a congenital bicuspid aortic valve is also at risk of bacterial endocarditis. All the congenital heart lesions associated with high-pressure jets, including ventricular septal defects and patent ductus arteriosus, carry a risk that the patient will develop infective endocarditis. Isolated atrial septal defects of the secundum type do not carry a risk, presumably due to the low-pressure blood flow across the defect.

Any form of prosthetic material inserted into the heart and exposed to the blood will promote thrombus formation and hence carries a risk of infective endocarditis. These include pacing catheters and Spitz-Holter valves in the right side of the heart, and prosthetic valves in the left side. All prosthetic valves in current use carry an appreciable and persistent risk of infection. With metal prostheses of the Starr ball-and-cage type, or the flat disc types, infection starts initially in the valve ring and extends outward into the adjacent myocardium. Vegetations are often not prominent but may extend as a pannus across the valve orifice. Dehiscence of the sutures anchoring the prosthesis may occur following destruction of the para-valve tissues.

Factors known to invoke bacteremia, and thus potentially cause bacterial endocarditis, include any form of urogenital instrumentation characteristically causing *S. fecalis* endocarditis; intravenous self-injection in drug addicts producing *Staph. aureus* endocarditis; and dental work causing *S. viridans* endocarditis.

The initial lesion is thought to be a small thrombus containing the organism of the endocardial surface of the cusp. As the lesions evolve, the thrombus grows in size and often extends along the cusp and onto adjacent endocardium. From the mitral valve, vegetations extend into the atria. Vegetations may spread from the aortic to the mitral valve and vice versa. The size and appearances of the vegetations vary markedly. Exuberant papillary vegetations are more common with staphylococcal infection of the mitral valve; aortic valve vegetations, even with the same organism, are smaller and more sessile. Sessile dome-shaped vegetations are produced by organisms of lower-grade virulence.

The underlying cusp tissue shows florid vascularization with an acute inflammatory infiltrate. Proliferation of fibroblasts at the base of the vegetation tends to wall off the infective lesion but seldom extends far into the thrombus; it simply pushes the whole mass outwards. Polymorphs are found in the thrombus but only in small numbers. Some organisms, particularly *Staph. aureus*, invoke striking fibrinoid necrosis of the underlying cusp collagen. With these organisms dissolution of the whole cusp structure leads to perforation and chordal rupture. It seems likely that once infection in a cusp is initiated, immune mechanisms cannot affect the sequestered organism; thus, in the past, when no bactericidal drugs were available, the outcome was inevitably fatal.

Treatment of the patient with bactericidal drugs results in micro-calcification of the bacterial colonies within the vegetations. Ultimately, sessile yellow calcified nodules are left on the cusp. Where tissue necrosis has occurred in the underlying valve tissue, treatment may not prevent cusp perforation and the development of significant regurgitation despite good control of the actual infection.

Complications of Bacterial Endocarditis

Patients with bacterial endocarditis may develop complications of cardiac failure, systemic emboli, and a range of immunologically determined phenomena resulting from circulating immune complexes. Cardiac failure in a patient with established bacterial endocarditis reflects various combinations of falling left ventricular contractility and increasing mitral or aortic regurgitation, as cusps perforate or chordae rupture. The decline in myocardial function is in part due to coronary micro-emboli, either as simple platelet thrombi or emboli containing the organism itself. Such emboli occur almost universally in patients with aortic valve endocarditis, due to the proximity of the vegetations to the coronary ostia. Superimposed immunological damage to small myo-

cardial vessels may also play a part in invoking myocardial damage. Cusp perforation and chordal rupture are associated with very rapid increases in volume load on the left ventricle, and this overload is poorly tolerated by the already damaged myocardium. This rapid deterioration is characteristic of infection with organisms such as *Staph. aureus* and is not instantly reversed by appropriate antibiotic therapy. Less virulent organisms produce simple fibrosis in the cusps, leading to a more gradual increase in regurgitation and slowly changing murmurs.

Embolic phenomena represent portions of thrombus, ranging from micro-fragments to masses 1 cm or more in diameter. They break free from the main mass of vegetations, and impact at any point in the systemic circulation. With the initiation of therapy the risk of embolism begins to fall steadily but does not disappear until the vegetations are organized and calcified throughout. Emboli containing virulent organisms may lead to an area of infarction which, becoming infected, leads to abscess fomation.

Emboli will occasionally cause an acute arteritis at the point of impaction and, particularly in the brain, produce aneurysms with a potential for rupture. Such mycotic aneurysms represent destruction of tissue by bacterial exotoxins when the embolus contains organisms; by proteases derived from polymorphs; and by immune complex-mediated damage when the embolus is itself sterile.

Immunological responses to circulating bacterial antigens leading to circulating immune complexes are responsible for a vasculitis in the skin, splinter hemorrhages, and a whole range of glomerular damage from focal to diffuse proliferative glomerulonephritis.

FUNGAL ENDOCARDITIS
(5.21 – 5.24)

Two groups contribute to those patients who develop fungal endocarditis: first, those with debilitating systemic disease in whom there has usually been depression of immunity by anti-neoplastic drugs or steroids; and second, those with prosthetic valves *in situ*. The common organisms include Candida, Aspergillus and Cryptococcus.

RICKETTSIAL ENDOCARDITIS
(5.25 – 5.27)

Endocarditis due to *Coxiella burneti* is now a well-recognized but rare disease. The disease usually results from pulmonary infection in patients with pre-existing valve lesions or prosthetic valves. Where the pulmonary phase is recognized it precedes the classic symptoms of an infective endocarditis by 6 to 18 months and the course of the cardiac lesion is very much of the 'chronic endocarditis' type. The vegetations are small and sessile and related to the contact lines of the valve cusps. Gross tissue destruction is unusual.

'CULTURE NEGATIVE' INFECTIVE ENDOCARDITIS

In recent years, patients have been recognized with all the clinical stigmata of infective endocarditis, yet positive blood culture cannot be obtained. Review of these cases suggest they fall into two groups, the more common being those who have received sub-therapeutic doses of antibiotics before blood culture was attempted. A rarer group are those infected with organisms which have specialized requirements for culture in the laboratory. It seems likely that so-called culture-negative infective endocarditis is really caused by an infectious agent, even if this cannot be established.

NON-BACTERIAL THROMBOTIC ENDOCARDITIS (NBTE) (5.28 – 5.31)

Perhaps no condition in the heart causes more confusion than NBTE since its macroscopic appearance may closely simulate true bacterial endocarditis. The synonyms in use for this condition include terminal, marantic, malignant or verrucous endocarditis, verrucous endocardiosis and endocarditis minima. In NBTE, the masses of thrombus attached to the valve cusps can range from sessile nodules only a few millimetres across, to exuberant masses up to 1cm in size. NBTE complicates many debilitating diseases but is seen most commonly in terminal malignancy, particularly with tumours of the lung, stomach, pancreas and ovary, although no primary tumour site is exempt from the phenomenon. One factor involved in the pathogenesis of NBTE is thought to be enhanced blood coagulation, since virtually identical valve lesions occur in known cases of disseminated intravascular coagulation. An additional factor may be mild valve swelling and endothelial damage invoked by the stress of severe illness. In most cases the condition is terminal and of no clinical consequence. A high proportion of cases coming to autopsy, however, can be shown to have had systemic emboli and, on occasions, the condition precedes death by a long enough period for emboli to be detected clinically. There are isolated case reports of patients who presented with systemic emboli some months before being found to have carcinoma. For the pathologist the difficulty is in distinguishing the condition from true infective endocarditis. Valuable pointers include the clinical history, the symmetrical involvement of the cusps, and the close relation of the vegetations to apposition lines of the cusps. Histologically, acute inflammation at the base of the thrombus is virtually absent, no colonies of organisms can be found, and culture of the vegetations yields no growth. Patients with NBTE who develop a bacteremia from any cause may be converted to true bacterial endocarditis.

References:

Bayliss R, Clarke C, Oakley C M, Somerville W and Whitefield A G W. The teeth and infective endocarditis. Br Heart J 1983; 50: 506-512.

Bayliss R, Clarke C, Oakley C M, Somerville W, Whitefield A G W and Young S E J. The microbiology and pathogenesis of infective endocarditis. Br Heart J 1983; 50: 513-519.

Bayliss R, Clarke C, Oakley C M, Somerville W, Whitefield A G W and Young S E J. The bowel, the genitourinary tract, and infective endocarditis. Br Heart J 1984; 51: 339-345.

Freedman L R and Valone J. Experimental infective endocarditis. Progress in Cardiovascular Disease 1979; 22: 169-180.

Invert T S A, Dismukes W E, Cobbs C G, Blackstone E H, Kirklin J W and Bergdahl L A L. Prosthetic valve endocarditis. Circulation 1984; 69: 223-232.

Phair J P and Clark J. Immunology of infective endocarditis. Progress in Cardiovascular Disease 1979; 22: 137-144.

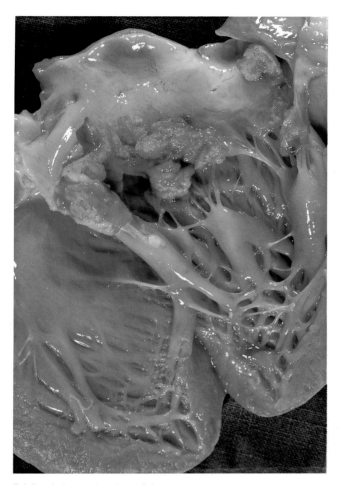

5.1 Staphylococcal endocarditis

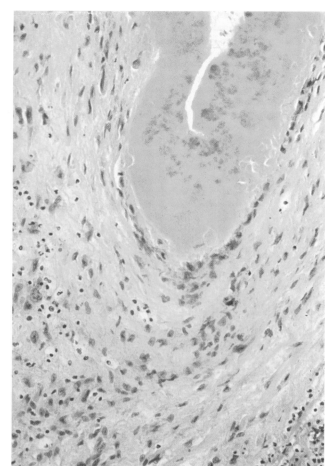

5.2 Staphylococcal endocarditis

5.1 Staphylococcal endocarditis on the mitral valve. The heart is opened to show the left atrium, left ventricle and the posterior cusp of the mitral valve. Vegetations in the form of red, irregular, cauliflower-like masses of thrombus cover the whole surface of the cusp and extend downwards onto the chordae.

5.2 Staphylococcal endocarditis: histology. Attached to the endocardial surface of the cusp is a mass of red-staining thrombus within which are numerous punctate purple-staining colonies of staphylococci. The underlying cusp tissue is hypercellular and contains numerous polymorphs. These, however, rarely extend far enough into the thrombus to reach the colonies of organisms. In addition to polymorphs the cusp tissue immediately beneath the thrombus contains macrophages, occasional giant cells and actively proliferating fibroblasts. Giant cells in the cusp are not uncommon in bacterial endocarditis and must not be mistaken as evidence of previous rheumatic disease.
x350 Hematoxylin and eosin.

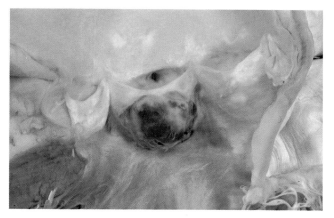

5.3 Staphylococcal endocarditis

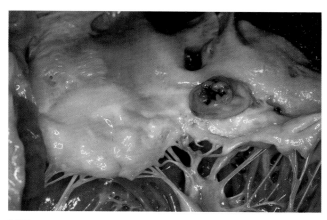

5.5 Bacterial endocarditis: floppy mitral valve

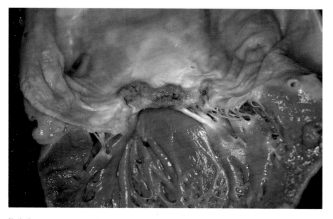

5.4 *Streptococcus viridans* endocarditis

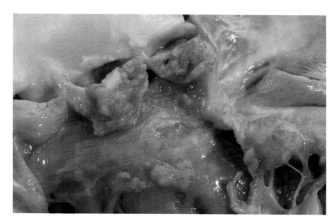

5.6 Bacterial endocarditis: hypertrophic cardiomyopathy

5.3   Acute staphylococcal endocarditis of the aortic valve. The patient, a woman aged 79, has a three-day history of pyrexia and rigors. She presented with a progressive hemiplegia due to a cerebral abscess from which the staphylococcus was grown. The vegetations on the valve are large red sessile masses but involve only one of the three aortic cusps. No evidence of pre-existing valve lesion is apparent. Very virulent organisms such as *Staph. aureus*, hemolytic streptococcus and pneumococcus may colonize valve cusps which are not clinically abnormal. With age, however, many aortic and mitral valves develop nodular thickening; thus all older subjects have valves which are to some extent abnormal and are at risk of endocarditis due to the very virulent organisms.

5.4   *Streptococcus viridans* infection of the mitral valve. The patient presented with systemic emboli and was previously known to have had chronic rheumatic mitral regurgitation. A sessile mass of dark thrombus lies on the lateral commissure of the mitral valve and projects up towards the atrium. The chordae of the valve are thickened from previous rheumatic disease.

5.5   Bacterial endocarditis in association with floppy mitral valve. The heart has been opened to show the left atrium and both cusps of the mitral valve. There is an oval mass of vegetations surrounding a perforation at the base of the posterior cusp. The anterior cusp has the ballooning deformity of the floppy mitral valve syndrome, suggesting pre-existing mitral regurgitation. The organism was *Staph. aureus*.

5.6   Bacterial endocarditis in hypertrophic cardiomyopathy. The left ventricular outflow has been opened through the aortic valve in a patient with hypertrophic cardiomyopathy who developed acute bacterial endocarditis. Vegetations cover the mitral valve and are present on the ventricular septum from where they have spread onto the aortic valve. The initial site of infection was probably the ventricular surface of the anterior cusp of the mitral valve, damaged by the impact with the septum that occurs in hypertrophic cardiomyopathy.

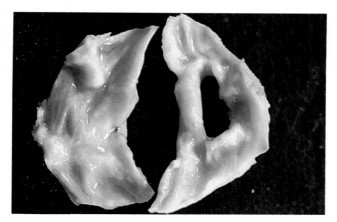

5.7 Bacterial endocarditis: aortic regurgitation

5.7 Aortic regurgitation in treated bacterial endocarditis.
Surgical specimen of bicuspid aortic valve excised for aortic regurgitation after a treated episode of endocarditis. One cusp has a clearly defined hole, with smooth edges, extending through the cusp body but all the vegetations have resolved. Such large well-defined perforations in the body of a cusp are always a consequence of bacterial infection.

5.8 Bacterial endocarditis in a patient with a right ventricular pacing wire.
The heart has been opened through the right atrium, tricuspid valve and right ventricle. A pacing wire crosses the tricuspid valve to be inserted in the apex of the right ventricle. Where the wire crosses the tricuspid valve it is covered by vegetations which extend into the ventricle. The wire was exteriorized to the skin from which site the patient developed staphylococcal sepsis, leading to septicemia and then to acute tricuspid endocarditis.

5.9 Bacterial endocarditis on a Starr mitral valve prosthesis.
The valve ring has been left intact and is viewed from the left atrium. Black silk sutures can be seen on the ring. Vegetations cover the valve ring and extend as a pannus out across the valve orifice, causing obstruction to flow and a situation hemodynamically akin to acute mitral valve stenosis.

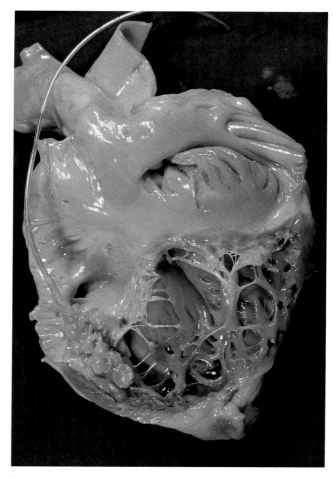

5.8 Bacterial endocarditis: pacing wire

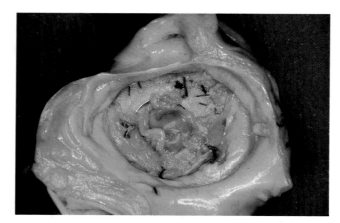

5.9 Bacterial endocarditis: Starr prosthesis

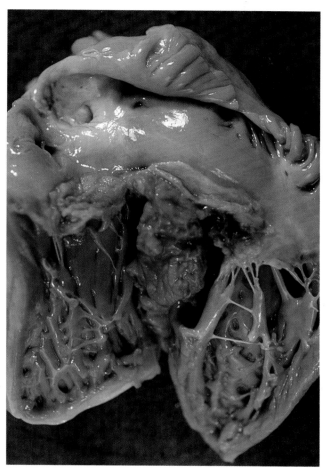

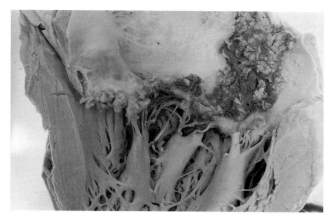

5.11 *Streptococcus viridans* endocarditis

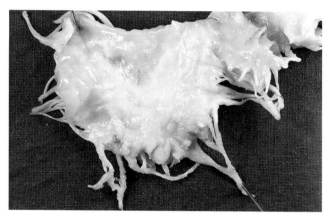

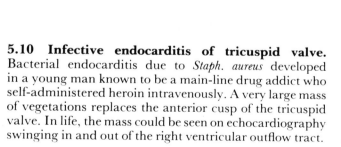

5.10 Infective endocarditis: tricuspid valve

5.12 Treated bacterial endocarditis

5.10 Infective endocarditis of tricuspid valve. Bacterial endocarditis due to *Staph. aureus* developed in a young man known to be a main-line drug addict who self-administered heroin intravenously. A very large mass of vegetations replaces the anterior cusp of the tricuspid valve. In life, the mass could be seen on echocardiography swinging in and out of the right ventricular outflow tract.

5.11 *Streptococcus viridans* endocarditis. The heart has been opened through the left atrium, ventricle and mitral valve and is from a patient with rheumatic mitral regurgitation. The specimen comes from a pathology museum from before the antibiotic era. Vegetations cover both anterior and posterior cusps and extend up into the left atrium on the endocardial surface. This spread into the atria was typical of untreated cases.

5.12 Treated bacterial endocarditis. Surgically-excised anterior cusp of mitral valve, removed after antibiotic treatment of acute bacterial endocarditis had left residual regurgitation. On the free edge of the cusp is a mass of sessile yellow calcified nodules. Such nodules arise from vegetations which calcify when the patient is treated with bactericidal drugs.

5.13 Myocardial damage in bacterial endocarditis.
A small artery within the myocardium contains a mass of embolic thrombus occluding the arterial lumen, but no organisms are present. From a patient with *Streptococcus viridans* endocarditis of the aortic valve.
x65 Hematoxylin and eosin.

5.14 Myocardial damage in bacterial endocarditis.
A small artery within the myocardium contains a mass of embolic thrombus which stains purple due to the presence of numerous organisms identified in life as *Staph. aureus*. The adjacent myocardium shows early infarction and is infiltrated by polymorphs and mononuclear cells. This is a septic embolus i.e. containing viable organisms in contrast to the bland sterile embolus in **5.13**.
x100 Hematoxylin and eosin.

5.15 Acute staphylococcal endocarditis.
Histological section across the vegetations on a valve cusp in acute staphylococcal endocarditis. The vegetations contain numerous basophilic punctate colonies of the organism. The connective tissue of the cusp underlying the vegetation has undergone necrosis and forms an acellular, slightly basophilic area. The necrosis is most likely mediated by proteases released from polymorphs. Such destruction is typical of highly virulent organisms.
x14 Hematoxylin and eosin.

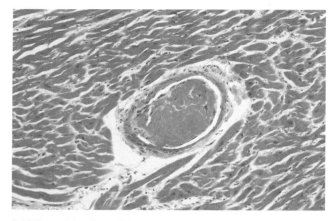

5.13 Bacterial endocarditis: myocardial damage

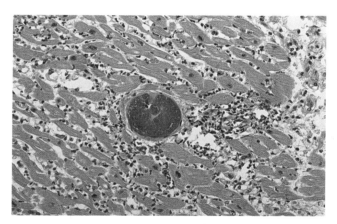

5.14 Bacterial endocarditis: myocardial damage

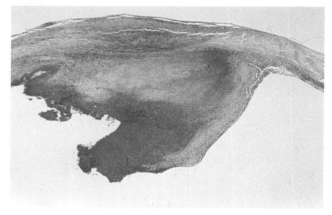

5.15 Acute Staphylococcal endocarditis

5.16 Cusp aneurysms following bacterial endocarditis. Surgically excised anterior cusp of the mitral valve following treatment of bacterial endocarditis, showing two cusp aneurysms. One has ruptured (blue marker). These aneurysms follow stretching, due to pressure from the blood, of damaged collagen in the cusp underlying the original vegetations. Having a mouth facing the high-pressure outflow tract of the left ventricle, they bulge toward the atrial surface and are almost always confined to the anterior cusp. Associated perforation is often present.

5.17 Para valve extension in bacterial endocarditis. Acute staphylococcal endocarditis in which there has been extension inward toward the valve ring to form a large mass which replaces the base of the aortic valve cusp. The mass consists largely of thrombus and its centre communicates with the cavity of the left ventricle by a small slit (arrow).

5.18 Para valve extension in bacterial endocarditis. Same case as **5.17** with the atrial septum viewed from the right side. Immediately anterior to the coronary sinus (C) are vegetations (arrows) on the endocardial surface where the mass of thrombus from the aortic root is eroding through into the right atrium. A few more days survival would have produced a left-to-right shunt. The atrio-ventricular node lies in this area and the patient developed heart block just before death.

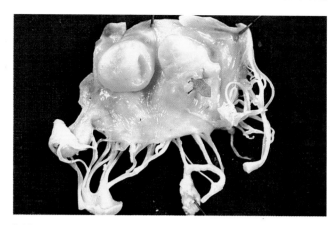

5.16 Bacterial endocarditis: cusp aneurysms

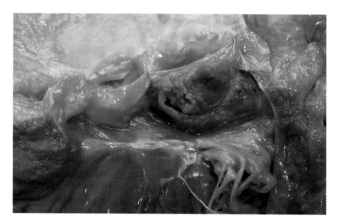

5.17 Bacterial endocarditis: para valve extension

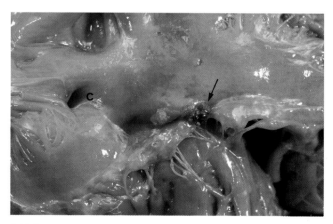

5.18 Bacterial endocarditis: para valve extension

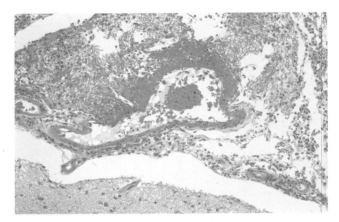

5.19 Bacterial endocarditis: cerebral arteritis

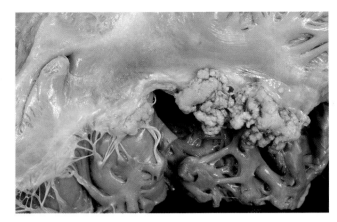

5.21 Fungal endocarditis: tricuspid valve

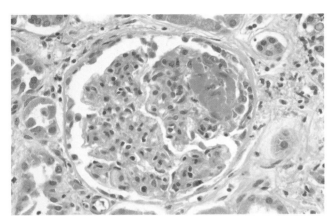

5.20 Bacterial endocarditis: focal glomerulonephritis

5.21 Fungal endocarditis on the tricuspid valve. The patient, who was on long term immunosuppression, developed oral candiasis following which blood cultures became positive for the fungus and vegetations on the tricuspid valve were demonstrated by echocardiography. The vegetations are large and yellow and cover the anterior cusp.

5.22 Fungal endocarditis on a Starr valve prosthesis. There is a Starr type prosthesis in the mitral valve which is viewed from the left atrium. The valve ball (poppet) is made of polypropylene. From the ring flat vegetations extend out across the valve opening but have not significantly impaired prosthetic function. In a patient with a prosthetic valve who is apparently well, sudden embolic phenomena are a common feature of fungal endocarditis. This patient died suddenly of main left coronary artery embolus. Infection starts in relation to the valve ring and extends into the orifice as vegetations. A para ring abscess may also form leading to dehiscence of the prosthesis.

5.19 Cerebral arteritis in bacterial endocarditis. Cerebral artery showing fibrinoid necrosis of a segment of the wall and a periadventitial acute inflammatory cell response in a patient with acute bacterial endocarditis. These mycotic aneurysms may rupture leading to intracranial hemorrhage.
x60 Hematoxylin and eosin.

5.23 Fungal endocarditis with coronary embolus. The main left coronary artery is virtually occluded by a mass of thrombus containing abundant magenta-stained fungal hyphae. The histology is from the same case as **5.22.** x35 Periodic acid - Schiff.

5.20 Glomerulonephritis in a patient with bacterial endocarditis. Glomerulus from a patient with bacterial endocarditis and hematuria. The glomerulus is hypercellular, and there is a focal area of bright red fibrinoid necrosis with adhesion to the capsule. This picture of focal glomerulonephritis is the most common histological response in bacterial endocarditis. Other rarer cases develop a diffuse proliferative glomerulonephritis which can lead to death from renal failure.
x500 Hematoxylin and eosin.

5.24 Fungal endocarditis. Tissue removed from valve ring of case in **5.22.** There is organizing thrombus containing abundant dark-staining fungal hyphae.
x225 Silver stain.

5.25 Rickettsial endocarditis. Histological section across the aortic valve cusp in a patient who developed regurgitation associated with extremely high titres of Coxiella antibodies. The cusp is hypercellular and there are collections of histiocytic cells (arrow).
x35 Hematoxylin and eosin.

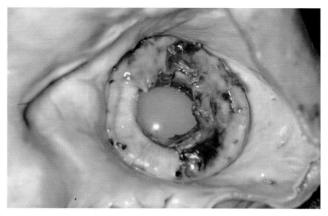

5.22 Fungal endocarditis: Starr valve

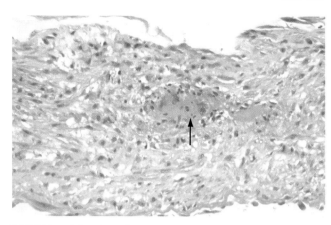

5.25 Rickettsial endocarditis

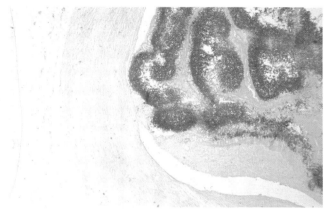

5.23 Fungal endocarditis: coronary embolus

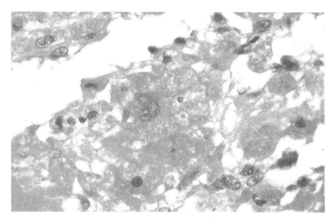

5.26 Rickettsial endocarditis

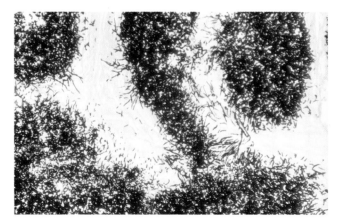

5.24 Fungal endocarditis

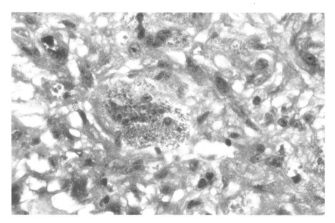

5.27 Rickettsial endocarditis

5.26 Rickettsial endocarditis. A higher-power view of the histiocytic cells shown in **5.25.** The cytoplasm contains numerous slightly basophilic organisms.
x625 Hematoxylin and eosin.

5.27 Rickettsial endocarditis. Intracellular rickettsial bodies in the cytoplasm of a histiocytic cell in the valve cusp.
x600 Giemsa.

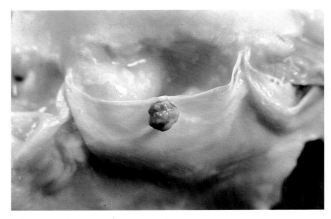

5.28 Non-bacterial thrombotic endocarditis

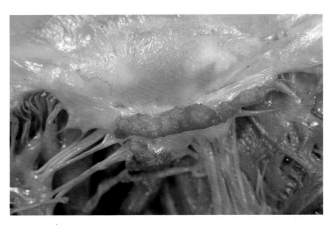

5.29 Non-bacterial thrombotic endocarditis

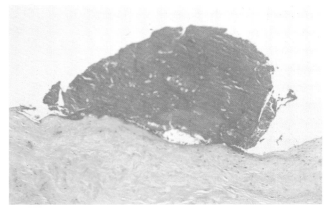

5.30 Non-bacterial thrombotic endocarditis

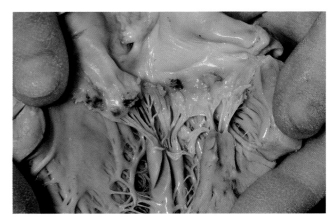

5.31 Diffuse intravascular coagulation

5.28   Non-bacterial thrombotic endocarditis. There is a small regular round mass of thrombus on the exact centre of the cusp of the aortic valve. This is typical of NBTE, atypical of true infective endocarditis.

5.29   Non-bacterial thrombotic endocarditis. There is a linear mass of thrombus along the apposition line of the anterior cusp of the mitral valve where it touches the posterior cusp in the closed position. Mitral valve NBTE may be very difficult to distinguish macroscopically from true infective endocarditis.

5.30   Non-bacterial thrombotic endocarditis. Histological section across the valve shown in **5.29**. A mass of red-staining thrombus adheres to the endothelial surface of the cusp; in contrast to bacterial endocarditis, no bacterial colonies are present and there is not an inflammatory response in the underlying cusp tissue. Histology is thus the safest way to separate NBTE from infective endocarditis.
x45 Hematoxylin and eosin.

5.31   Diffuse intravascular coagulation. Strands and fronds of thrombotic material are present along the apposition line of the mitral valve cusps in a child dying of diffuse intravascular coagulation. This could be regarded as one form of NBTE.

CHAPTER 6

Ischemic Heart Disease

Ischemic heart disease is the term applied to the effects of a reduction or cessation of the blood supply to the myocardium. In the vast majority of patients the impairment of blood flow is due to the disease known as atheroma (atherosclerosis). There are rare conditions such as coronary emboli, coronary arteritis or anomalous origins of a coronary artery which can also lead to ischemic damage to the myocardium but for practical purposes the term ischemic heart disease is synonymous with coronary atheroma.

Some degree of coronary atheroma is almost inevitable in individuals living in Western populations but such subjects are not regarded as suffering from ischemic heart disease until clinical symptoms or myocardial damage occurs.

ATHEROMA
(6.1 – 6.8)

Atherosclerosis (atheroma) can be defined as a disease of large and medium arteries in which there is focal proliferation of smooth muscle cells and accumulation of lipid within the intima. A striking feature is the focal distribution of the lesions, known as 'plaques', within the intima.

When the intimal surface of an involved artery such as the aorta is examined by the naked eye, several distinct lesions may be recognized, all of which are encompassed within the generic term atheroma.

Simple fatty streaks or dots are barely raised above the surface while the raised plaque forms a distinct hump. The complicated plaque has ulcerated, with thrombus forming on the surface. It is tempting to suppose that these lesions develop sequentially. There is, however, strong epidemiological evidence that the simple fatty streak occurs in all geographic populations, and is not dependent on an appreciable incidence of clinically expressed ischemic disease. This suggests that many fatty streaks are static lesions which do not evolve. It is clear that the complication of thrombosis, leading directly or indirectly to clinical symptoms of atheroma, develop on the raised plaque. Yet there are many individuals who have raised plaques and who do not develop thrombosis. This fact has led to the view that there are two stages in the development of ischemic heart disease: the first simply produces plaques; the second produces thrombosis and symptoms.

It is beyond the scope of an atlas to review the pathogenesis of atheroma. It must suffice to say that atheroma has two essential elements, smooth muscle proliferation and lipid accumulation. The two processes are not directly

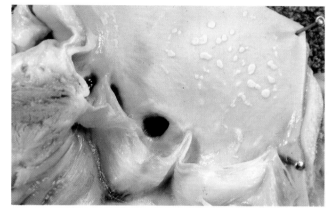

6.1 Fatty dots

6.1   Fatty dots. This picture shows punctate deposits of lipid within the intima. These fatty dots are common in the ascending aorta, just above the aortic valve.

linked. Even in the same individual there are atheromatous plaques with very different proportions of lipid to smooth muscle. The hard pearly plaque has virtually no lipid; the soft plaque has a vast central pool of lipid with minimal connective tissue. In general, the more lipid present, the more likely are thrombotic complications to occur. It should be stressed that the histological variation in plaques is vast, but the basic theme of smooth muscle proliferation and lipid accumulation runs through them all. The current trend of research into the early pathogenesis of atheroma as a disease process stresses the role of endothelial cell damage as the early initiating event. This allows reaction of platelets with the intima, the release of platelet mitogen factors, resulting in smooth muscle proliferation. Lipid passes through the damaged endothelial cells from the plasma to accumulate in the intima.

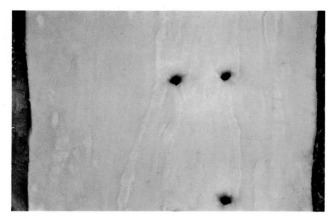

6.2 Fatty streaks

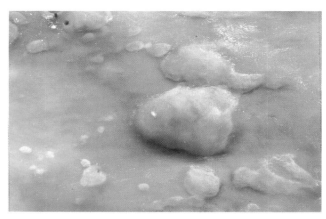

6.4 Raised plaque

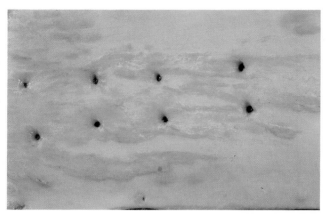

6.3 Fatty streaks

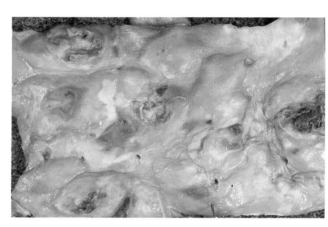

6.5 Complicated plaques

6.2 Fatty streaks. Here fatty streaks are seen as linear deposits of lipid within the intima. These fatty streaks are common in the descending aorta. Fatty dots and fatty streaks are the earliest lesions of atheroma.

6.3 Fatty streaks. The aorta has been immersed in Sudan stain. This stains the lipid present in the intima as bright red. In the picture are shown a mixture of fatty streaks and fatty dots in the descending aorta.

6.4 Raised plaque. In this picture two raised plaques are seen rising, dome-shaped, above the intimal surface. These plaques appear white rather than yellow because they have a fibrous cap. Also in the picture, lower left, are some fatty dots.

6.5 Complicated plaques. On the intimal surface of the abdominal aorta are numerous raised plaques many of which have ulcerated and have thrombus on the intimal surface.

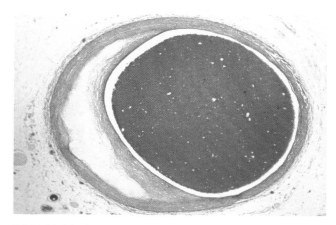

6.6 Lipid-rich plaque

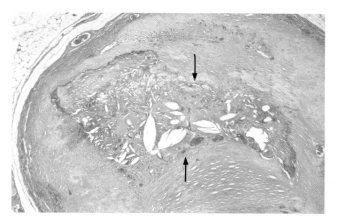

6.7 Lipid in a plaque

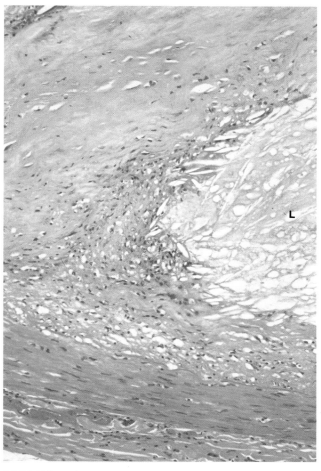

6.8 Lipid in a plaque

6.6   Simple lipid-rich atheromatous plaque. Transverse histological section of a simple atheromatous plaque in a coronary artery which was perfused post mortem with a gelatin-barium suspension. The lumen of the artery is distended by the injected material and is thus round. The plaque is a crescent-shaped area of intimal thickening with a clear zone which was occupied by lipid before the tissues were prepared for histology. The plaque is convex, bulging into the media rather than inward toward the lumen which remains circular. The term 'raised plaque' is thus a misnomer; the appearance is an artefact produced by opening the artery longitudinally. The lipid within the plaque is separated from the lumen by an intact cap of fibrous tissue.
x20 Elastic-hematoxylin and eosin.

6.7   Lipid within an atheromatous plaque. The intima is thickened by fibrous tissue within which is contained a 'pool' of lipid (arrows). Cholesterol crystals recognizable as boat or needle-shaped open spaces are present.
x50 Hematoxylin and eosin.

6.8   Lipid within an atheromatous plaque. Histological section of part of an atheromatous plaque. The centre of the plaque is acellular, with the lipid (L) lying free and as cholesterol clefts. At the margin of this lipid-filled pool are foam and giant cells containing intracellular lipid.
x225 Hematoxylin and eosin.

References:

Woolf N. Pathology of Atherosclerosis. London: Butterworths 1982.

Woolf N ed. Biology and Pathology of the Vessel Wall. A Modern Appraisal. Eastbourne and New York: Praeger 1983.

MYOCARDIAL METABOLISM
AND ENERGY PRODUCTION

The myocardium is unique in that there is an inherent need for constant high levels of energy production interspersed with bursts of physical exercise in which energy production must further increase. Within myocardial cells the mitochondria metabolize glucose, lactate and fatty acids to constantly produce the high energy phosphates, adenosine triphosphate (ATP) and creatinine phosphate. Energy production is aerobic and dependent on oxygen and thus on blood supply. The inherent high oxygen demand of the myocardium is reflected in very low venous O_2 saturation; coronary sinus blood oxygen saturation is 25-35% in contrast to 70% in the venous blood draining skeletal muscle. The implication of the high extraction rate of O_2 in the myocardium is that on exercise the increased oxygen demand cannot be met by increased extraction, but must be largely met by increasing blood flow.

Energy generated within the myocardial cell is predominantly used for contraction; ATP is split at the myofibrils by myosin ATPase and with Ca^{++} invokes sliding of the actin and myosin filaments to generate contraction. A minor, but significant, proportion of energy production is used to maintain membrane integrity both within the cell and in relation to the external environment.

If O_2 supply falls below that required to maintain myofibrillary contraction for a very short period glycogen is metabolized in anaerobic energy production following which lactate accumulates, ATP levels fall and intracellular pH rises. The initial reversible phase of ischemia is associated with the genesis of anginal pain by unknown mechanisms. Cessation of blood flow for over 10-15 minutes leads to irreversible cell damage. ATP levels fall to virtually zero within the cell and contraction ceases. As membrane integrity is lost, calcium ions enter the cell and accumulate within mitochondria. Cell membrane damage allows K^+ ions and intracellular enzymes to leave the cell. This sequence of irreversible changes is the cellular basis of myocardial infarction.

NORMAL INTRAMYOCARDIAL
BLOOD FLOW

Intramyocardial blood flow cannot occur in systole due to the compressive effect on the blood vessels of myocardial contraction. It is only the epicardial coronary arteries that fill in systole and as intramyocardial pressure falls in diastole blood from the epicardial arteries and aortic root

enters the myocardium. Intramyocardial flow is thus entirely a diastolic phenomenon dependent on the pressure gradient in diastole between the aortic root and the left ventricular cavity. Intramyocardial blood flow can be reduced by tachycardia which shortens diastole more than systole and by a fall in aortic root pressure as in shock or by a rise of left ventricular diastolic pressure as in aortic valve stenosis. All these factors have a disproportionate effect in reducing blood flow to the subendocardial as compared to the subpericardial muscle layer particularly when ventricular wall thickness is increased as in pressure overload hypertrophy.

A further factor determining the pattern of ischemic myocardial damage is that the blood supply to the myocardium is regional. This implies that each major arterial branch supplies a specific portion of myocardial muscle and in terms of function the degree of overlap from neighbouring arteries is minimal.

EXPERIMENTAL
MYOCARDIAL INFARCTION

Ligation of a coronary artery in the dog leads to infarction of the segment of myocardium supplied by that artery. The time sequences relating the duration of occlusion to the necrosis induced can be studied and may have close analogies to human coronary artery disease.

Biochemical changes within the myocardial cells begin within a minute but the injury is reversible for at least 15 minutes as judged by the prevention of necrosis if the ligature is removed. If flow is occluded for 40 minutes, infarction is inevitable even if flow is restored. From 40 minutes up to 3 hours of occlusion the infarct is confined to the subendocardial zone, 6 hours of occlusion leads to a full thickness (transmural) infarction. The infarct thus spreads through the ventricular wall over a 6-hour period but the lateral margins are established by 40 minutes of occlusion emphasizing the regional nature of coronary arterial blood supply.

PATHOLOGICAL BASIS
OF ISCHEMIC SYNDROMES
IN MAN
(6.9 – 6.40)

Angina represents pain arising in myocardial tissue which is suffering reversible ischemic changes. Patients with angina fall into two groups; those in whom the pain is predictable being invoked by a fixed level of exercise are classified as stable in type. The other group with unstable angina have pain whose onset is unpredictable and often occurs at rest.

STABLE ANGINA
(6.9 – 6.20)

Stable angina is due to fixed arterial obstruction which limits any increase in coronary blood flow. It is usually regarded that stenosis of at least 75% by cross sectional area (50% by diameter) is required to produce angina on exercise.

Prognosis in an individual patient can be crudely assessed by whether one, two or three of the major coronary arteries have stenotic segments of this degree. Stenosis of the main stem of the left coronary artery is also regarded as a grave prognostic indicator. There is a considerable range in the histological appearances of stenotic arterial lesions. The major variations arise from permutations of two pairs of characteristics. The atheromatous plaque may be concentric, that is, involve the whole circumference of the intima; or eccentric, that is, involve only one segment of the intima. In the latter case there is a segment of arterial wall with normal medial muscle partially surrounding the residual lumen. The atheromatous plaque may be composed predominantly of fibromuscular intimal proliferation containing varying amounts of intracellular lipid or contain within the intima a pool of free extracellular lipid. This pool contains cholesterol and its esters recognizable as needle or boat-shaped crystals. The majority of these plaques also contain ceroid pigment which is lipid droplets with a protein coat insoluble in fat solvents. The bright yellow colour of the lipid pool is due to carotenoid pigment rather than lipid itself. In arteries distended at physiological pressures the lumen is roughly circular in shape, and the slit and star shapes so frequently illustrated are artefacts of collapsed vessels. In distended arteries the plaque bulges outward into the media and has usually broken the internal elastic lamina. The medial muscle vanishes behind such plaques and there is an adventitial chronic inflammatory response which may include cells in response to released lipid. These patients may develop autoantibodies to lipoprotein complexes.

A high proportion of patients with stable angina also have arterial segments in which the original lumen is blocked by connective tissue within which more than one new vascular channel has developed. This pattern is regarded as resulting from organization and recanalization of a previous episode of occlusive thrombosis. While such segments of recanalization are common in patients with a previous history of myocardial infarction, they are also

found in over 60% of patients with angina who do not have previous infarction. This fact underlines that many occlusive thrombi do not lead to infarction and that thrombosis is an important cause of clinical progression in patients with stable angina.

Calcification is always described as one of the major complications of atheroma and is important since it hinders dissection by the surgeon or pathologist. Calcification, however, is not directly related to the degree of stenosis and many patients over 75 years of age have widely patent but calcified arteries. The calcification is within the intima and medial calcification analogous to Monckeberg's disease of the lower limb is rare in the coronary arteries.

UNSTABLE ANGINA
(6.10, 6.15, 6.21 – 6.27)

The hallmark of unstable angina is the unpredictable onset of the pain which is not related to exercise. The pain reflects reversible myocardial ischemia invoked by a variation in the cross-sectional area of some segments of stenosis. The name dynamic stenosis has been given to this process. There is considerable clinical and morphological evidence to suggest that the pathophysiological basis of unstable angina is heterogeneous. One group of patients have episodes of pain which are increasing in severity, duration and frequency, and culminate in sudden death or acute myocardial infarction, or the patient suddenly recovers from what is known as crescendo angina. Other patients have episodic rest pain which is constant in character over long periods and associated with concomitant exercise induced angina.

Two separate pathophysiological mechanisms have been described. In one there is marked variation in vasomotor tone at arterial segments in which high grade stenosis exists due to an eccentric plaque. Such plaques allow the residual lumen to have at least part of its circumference occupied by normal medial muscle. Contraction of this muscle alters the calibre of the already stenotic arterial segment. There is clinical evidence that all eccentric plaques are associated with variation in lumen diameter when challenged by vasoconstrictor drugs, but patients with unstable angina develop spontaneous spasm for unknown reasons. A minority of patients with atheroma have eccentric plaques as the predominant form and may be particularly prone to develop unstable angina. There is a rare form of unstable angina (variant type) particularly found in women in which spasm occurs in normal coronary arteries independent of atheromatous disease.

The second mechanism for dynamic stenosis is concerned with plaques that are undergoing fissuring or rupture in consequence of which mural thrombus develops on the intimal surface. This process is the usual basis of the crescendo type of unstable angina. Plaques which are undergoing fissuring can be detected in life by coronary arteriography as segments of stenosis with very irregular or overhanging edges.

Plaques which are undergoing fissuring develop mural thrombus which waxes and wanes in size and thus in the degree of obstruction that is caused. Episodes of pain also reflect multiple small emboli, consisting predominantly of platelets, which impact in the small vessels of the myocardium downstream of fissured plaques. Multiple microscopic foci of necrosis develop particularly in the subpericardial zone of the myocardium.

SUDDEN DEATH DUE TO ISCHEMIC HEART DISEASE (6.21 – 6.27)

Clinical studies of patients rescued from 'sudden death' by emergency resuscitation teams have shown that the vast majority of such episodes are due to the onset of ventricular fibrillation, that up to 50% of the patients have prodomal symptoms of chest pain in the preceding week and that in 'survivors' acute myocardial infarction occurs only in a minority of 20-30%. Post mortem coronary angiography has demonstrated that virtually all patients dying suddenly of ischemic heart disease have plaques undergoing fissuring and over which mural thrombus is forming. Only a minority, however, have thrombi large enough to be occlusive and prevent distal flow in the vessel. It is this minority of patients who would be likely to develop infarction had they lived. In those with mural non-occlusive thrombosis there is, as in unstable angina, an approximately 30% incidence of demonstrable platelet micro-emboli in the myocardium at autopsy. The pathology of sudden ischemic death is therefore one of 'dynamic stenosis' due to mural thrombosis identical to one form of unstable angina.

ACUTE MYOCARDIAL INFARCTION (6.28 – 6.40)

The term myocardial infarction is applied correctly to necrosis of myocardial cells mediated by cessation, reduction or interference with their blood supply. This simple definition takes no account of the different patterns of necrosis that occur and which are mediated by different pathophysiological mechanisms. Few subjects have invoked more fruitless controversy among pathologists than the pathogenesis of acute infarction largely created by a failure to distinguish the different types.

It is of great importance to distinguish the pattern of myocardial necrosis in particular whether the infarction is regional or more generalized. The classification is made far more easily if a complete cross-section of the ventricles in the short axis is stained to demonstrate enzyme activity. This technique allows large areas of necrosis to be identified macroscopically by their enzyme loss.

The major distinction which has to be made is between areas of infarction which are regional, i.e. in the territory supplied by one major coronary artery branch and those which are diffuse. It is regional infarction which is related to obstruction to flow in the artery subtending the area of necrosis. In very rare instances the artery may be morphologically normal and coronary artery spasm must be held to be the cause. Although impossible to prove at autopsy, clinical evidence firmly suggests that this phenomenon exists. The vast majority of acute regional infarcts, however, can be related to thrombi occurring on atheromatous plaques which are undergoing fissuring. The pathological controversies over whether this thrombosis had to be occlusive to cause infarction have largely been resolved by clinical angiography within the first four hours after the onset of pain. Such studies have shown that within the first hour over 90% of arteries supplying an acute regional infarction are occluded. Over the succeeding hours a proportion of these vessels re-open spontaneously but the flow can be restored in the majority by intra-coronary infusion of fibrinolytic agents. Following restoration of blood flow a high grade stenosis with ragged outlines is revealed and filling defects within the contrast media suggest that it is thrombus that is being lysed. This clinical data confirms the pathological view that many regional infarcts are related to fissured plaques and also shows that thrombosis is a very dynamic process. It is a nonsense for pathologists to believe that they can have valid views at autopsy on the presence or absence of occlusive thrombi twenty-four hours before the patient died. Nevertheless, the majority of patients with full thickness transmural regional infarction do have, at autopsy, a totally occluded artery. Studies using radiolabelled fibrinogen given within the first hour of pain have shown that the thrombus seen at autopsy has a radionegative proximal portion over a fissured plaque and a radiolabelled distal tail. Such work confirms that thrombi are formed before infarction develops but continue to propagate distally over many hours. It is likely that such distal propagation is linked to large infarcts and to cardiogenic shock, and is more common in fatal than non-fatal infarction.

Regional subendocardial infarction, that is, where the necrosis does not extend through the full thickness of the ventricular wall, is far less consistently associated with a completely occluded artery. This form of infarction is regarded either as arising following occlusions which re-open due to spontaneous fibrinolysis within the period of 40 minutes to 3 hours, thus restoring flow before the infarct has become transmural, or due to the previous establishment of collateral flow to the subpericardial zone.

Diffuse forms of necrosis are related to the problems of overall myocardial perfusion rather than to thrombosis in one artery. Such infarction ranges from necrosis confined to the centres of the papillary muscles, to loss of the inner third of the ventricular wall throughout the whole circumference of the left ventricle. The most severe forms often have focal necrosis in right ventricular muscle. Diffuse myocardial necrosis may occur totally independent of coronary atheroma, and is a reflection of low aortic diastolic pressure as in shock, or high diastolic pressure in the left ventricle as in cardiac failure due to aortic valve disease. Thick-walled or dilated left ventricles are particularly prone to develop subendocardial necrosis. Any patient who has severe and prolonged left ventricular failure may develop this form of diffuse subendocardial necrosis, and it is less confusing to use this name than to describe the lesion as an infarct. Hearts from patients with severe coronary artery disease on whom macroscopic enzyme studies are normal, will often show multifocal microscopic foci of necrosis. This form of necrosis cannot be linked to any particular mechanism and reflects many different processes including platelet emboli, high grade coronary stenosis and falling overall myocardial perfusion. Identical microscopic foci occur in conditions as diverse as severe left ventricular hypertrophy, hypokalemia and high levels of circulating catecholamines.

References:

Davies M J, Fulton W F M and Robertson W B. The relation of coronary thrombosis to ischemic myocardial necrosis. J Pathol 1979; 127: 99-110.

Davies M J and Thomas T. The pathological basis and microanatomy of occlusive thrombus formation in human coronary arteries. Philosophical Transactions of the Royal Society of London 1981; 294: 225-229.

Davies M J, Thomas A C. Plaque fissuring – the cause of acute myocardial infarction, sudden ischemic death and crescendo angina. Br Heart J 1985; 53: 363-373.

Dewood M A, Spores J, Notske R. Prevalence of total coronary occlusion during the early hours of transmural myocardial infarction. N England J Med 1980; 303: 897-902.

Falk E. Plaque rupture with severe pre-existing stenosis precipitating coronary thrombosis. Characteristics of coronary atherosclerotic plaque underlying fatal occlusive thrombi. Br Heart J 1983; 50: 127-134.

Falk E. Unstable angina with fatal outcome: dynamic coronary thrombosis leading to infarction and/or sudden death. Circulation 1985; 71: 699-708.

Levin D C, Fallon J T. Significance of the angiographic morphology of localized coronary stenoses: histopathologic correlations. Circulation 1982; 66: 316-320.

Lichtlen P R, Rafflenbeul W, Freudenberg H. Pathoanatomy and function of coronary obstructions leading to unstable angina pectoris: anatomical and angiographic studies. In Hugenholz P G, Goldman B S eds., Unstable Angina. Stuttgart: Shattauer, 1985: 81-94.

Reimer K A, Jennings R B. The wavefront phenomenon of ischemic cell death. II Transmural progression of necrosis within the framework of ischemic bed size (myocardium at risk) and collateral flow. Laboratory Investigation 1979; 40: 633-644.

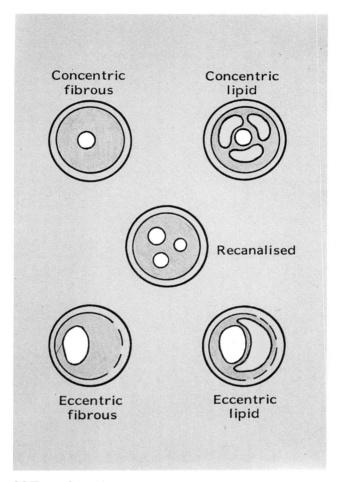

6.9 Types of stenosis

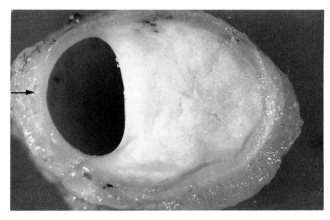

6.10 Eccentric plaque: stenosis

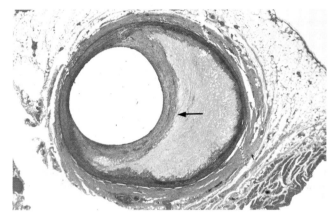

6.11 Eccentric lipid-rich plaque

6.9 Morphological types of coronary stenosis. In this diagram lipid is represented as yellow, fibrous tissue as grey, the residual lumen remaining white. Stenoses can be divided into four types, concentric fibrous, concentric lipid, eccentric fibrous and eccentric lipid, depending on the situation of the plaque and whether it has a lipid pool.

6.10 Eccentric plaque causing stenosis. This artery has been fixed by distention at 120mm Hg with formal saline. The plaque is eccentric, displacing the lumen from the mid-line. Opposite the plaque there is a segment of normal artery wall (arrow). It is plaques of this type that retain the potential for medial muscle contraction to alter the cross-sectional area of the lumen. Dissecting Microscope appearance.

6.11 Eccentric lipid rich plaque. The artery has been fixed by distention; the lumen is round and there is an eccentric plaque occupying one segment of the circumference of the artery. The eccentric nature of the plaque leaves an arc of normal media. The plaque contains a crescentic pale area where lipid was present. This lipid pool is separated from the lumen by a thin cap of fibrous tissue (arrow).
x25 Elastic-hematoxylin and eosin.

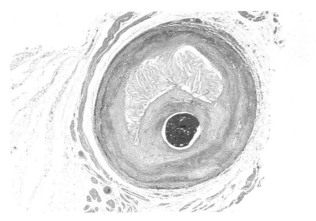

6.12 Atheroma: high grade stenosis

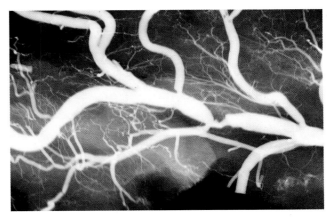

6.14 High grade stenosis: arteriogram

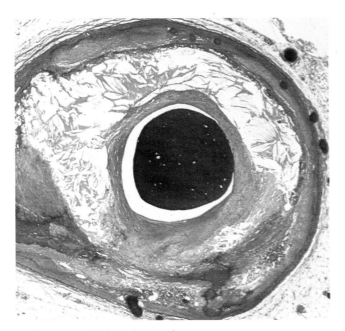

6.13 Atheroma: high grade stenosis

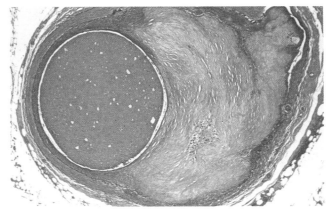

6.15 Eccentric plaque: stenosis

6.12   Coronary atheroma causing high grade stenosis. Severe coronary artery stenosis caused by almost concentric intimal thickening within which there are large amounts of extracellular lipid. The lumen is circular but set slightly off-centre from the vessel. This is a lipid-rich lesion.
x35 Elastic-hematoxylin and eosin.

6.13   Coronary atheroma causing high grade stenosis. There is severe stenosis due to concentric thickening. Within the intima a large pool of lipid extends almost around the whole circumference of the artery. Such stenoses have no potential for variation in the lumen cross-sectional area.
x25 Elastic-hematoxylin and eosin.

6.14   Arteriographic appearance of fixed stenosis. In this post mortem angiogram there is a single area of high grade stenosis with smooth edges in the right coronary artery. The histology of this lesion is shown in **6.13**. Smooth outlines not associated with intraluminal filling defects are the appearances on angiography of stable plaques which are not undergoing any acute change and are designated as being of Type I.

6.15   Stenosis due to an eccentric fibrous plaque. The stenosis is caused by eccentric intimal thickening which is predominantly fibrous without a lipid pool. A segment of normal media remains and variation in smooth muscle tone could lead to significant alterations in the cross-sectional area of the lumen.
x30 Elastic-hematoxylin and eosin.

6.16 Coronary atheroma causing high grade stenosis. Severe coronary artery stenosis due to concentric intimal thickening which is predominantly collagenous and contains minimal lipid. The arterial lumen is central. This is a purely fibrous lesion.
x25 Elastic-hematoxylin and eosin.

6.17 Coronary atheroma causing high grade stenosis. Very severe coronary artery stenosis caused by intimal thickening in which there is minimal lipid deposition. The collagenous thickening is in two distinct layers which have slightly different staining properties.
x13 Elastic-hematoxylin and eosin.

6.18 Coronary atheroma causing high grade stenosis. Severe stenosis of a small coronary artery due to massive eccentric intimal thickening which contains numerous lipid-filled histiocytes but relatively little collagen or free cholesterol. This form of lipid deposition is common in diabetes and hyperlipidemic states in man. It is also seen in induced hypercholesterolemia in experimental animals. It characteristically involves somewhat smaller vessels than the usual form of atheroma.
x25 Hematoxylin and eosin.

6.19 Recanalization pattern in coronary atheroma. Cross-section of coronary artery stenosis showing many new channels containing angiographic media within the original vessel lumen. Lipid is not present. This appearance is usually the result of organization of a propagation thrombus which was occluding a vessel distal to an athertomatous plaque.
x25 Hematoxylin and eosin.

6.19a Coronary atheroma: recanalization. In the post mortem angiogram the presence of several channels within the original lumen can be recognized.

6.20 Coronary atheroma: calcification. Calcification in the intima due to atheroma. There is eccentric fibrous thickening of the intima. Deep in the fibrous tissue there are many cholesterol clefts and an irregular circular area of deeper-staining basophilic calcification (arrows).
x40 Elastic-hematoxylin and eosin.

6.20a Coronary atheroma: calcification. In this plain AP X ray of the heart calcification can be seen to outline the main coronary arteries.

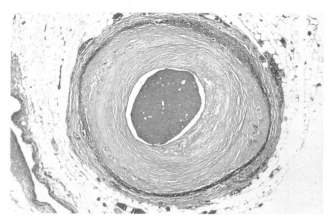

6.16 Atheroma: high grade stenosis

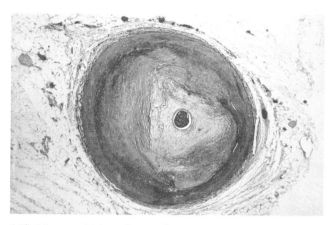

6.17 Atheroma: high grade stenosis

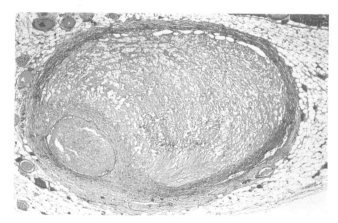

6.18 Atheroma: high grade stenosis

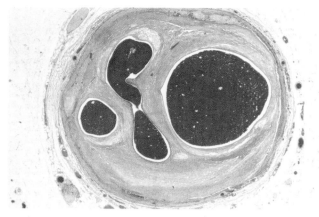

6.19 Atheroma: recanalization

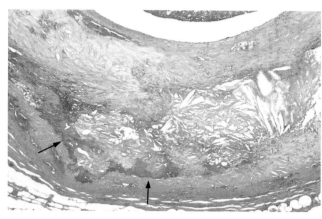

6.20 Atheroma: calcification

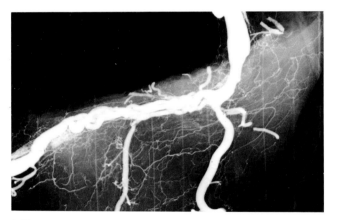

6.19a Coronary atheroma: recanalization

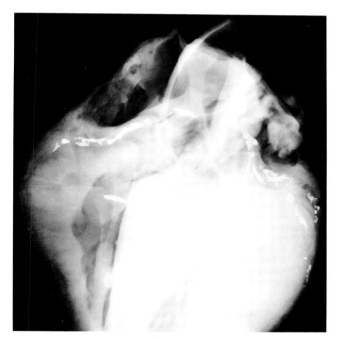

6.20a Coronary atheroma: calcification

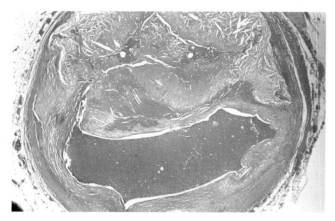

6.21 Fissuring of plaque

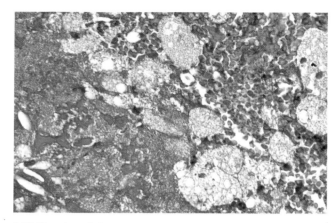

6.22 Fissuring of plaque

6.21 Fissuring of atheromatous plaque. Transverse section of plaque within which extensive thrombus containing a considerable number of red cells has formed. A fissure can be traced from the lumen down into the plaque. Injection medium is also present deep in the plaque. The majority of so-called intra-plaque hemorrhages are due to the same process of fissuring with a communication to the lumen. Unless serial sections are used, however, the existence of this communication may not be noted.
x25 Elastic-hematoxylin and eosin.

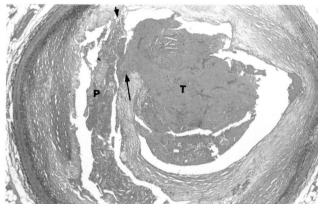

6.23 Fissuring of plaque

6.22 Fissuring of atheromatous plaque. Higher-power view of the depths of the plaque shown in **6.21**. Within the plaque there are red cells (stained orange), platelets (punctate blue material), fibrin (red), and foamy histiocytic cells. The modified Picro-Mallory stain used here is ideal for differentiating the components of a thrombus.
x375 Picro-Mallory trichrome.

6.23 Fissuring of atheromatous plaque. There is a fissure in the cap of a plaque (arrows). Thrombus within the plaque (P) protrudes through the fissure to project into the lumen (T) of the artery which contains angiographic material. The artery is not totally occluded.
x30 Elastic-hematoxylin and eosin.

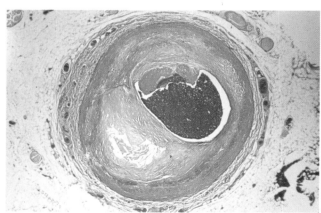

6.24 Thrombosis on a plaque

6.24 Thrombosis on an atheromatous plaque. Transverse section of an atheromatous plaque in a coronary artery. The lumen of the artery contains post-mortem angiographic medium. There is an eccentric area of intimal thickening with a lipid pool. At one edge of the plaque, bright red thrombus has been deposited on the endothelial surface, but in this section the fibrous cap of the plaque is intact. The thrombus shown here would be designated as mural because the lumen is not occluded.
x16 Elastic-hematoxylin and eosin.

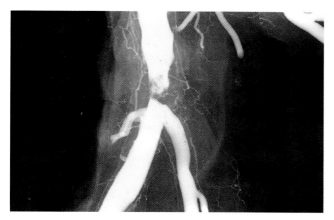

6.25 Fissuring of plaque: angiogram

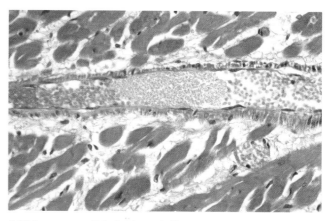

6.26 Intramyocardial platelet emboli

6.25 Coronary angiogram illustrating a fissured plaque. Fissured plaques with overlying mural thrombus can be detected in both post-mortem and clinical angiograms by the sharp acute edges of the stenotic segment and by the intraluminal filling defect. These appearances are designated as Type II lesions to distinguish them from the smooth indentations produced by stable plaques and known as Type I lesions.

6.26 Intramyocardial platelet emboli. A small artery is seen in longitudinal section. Within the artery is a mass consisting entirely of purple staining platelets. On either side of the platelet plug the vessel contains red cells stained yellow. The patient had unstable angina and died suddenly. The coronary artery supplying this segment of myocardium contained a fissured plaque with overlying mural thrombus.
x375 Picro-Mallory trichrome.

6.27 Intramyocardial platelet emboli. A small intramyocardial artery seen in cross-section is completely blocked by a mass of purple staining platelets with a few strands of red staining fibrin. This small embolus arose from more proximal mural thrombus.
x425 Picro-Mallory trichrome.

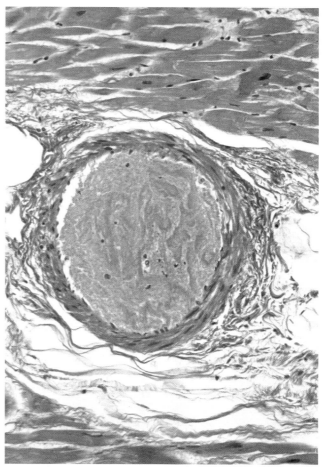

6.27 Intramyocardial platelet emboli

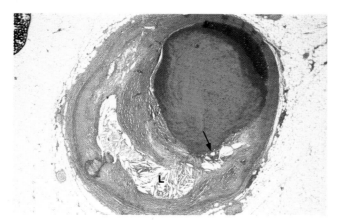

6.28 Coronary thrombosis

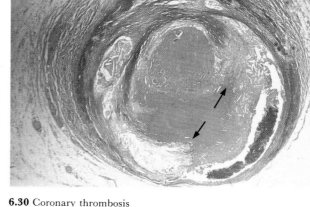

6.30 Coronary thrombosis

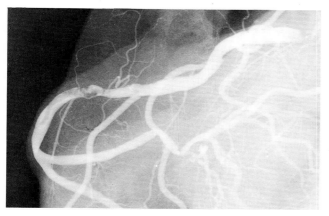

6.29 Coronary thrombosis

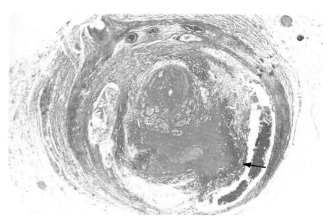

6.31 Coronary thrombosis

6.28 Coronary thrombosis. Transverse section of a coronary artery (left anterior descending) from a patient dying of acute anterior myocardial infarction. There is intimal thickening due to an atheromatous plaque with a large lipid (L) pool. The lumen is almost totally occluded by a large mass of red-staining fibrin-rich thrombus, although some post-mortem angiographic medium has passed over the thrombus where it has retracted from the vessel wall. At one point the plaque cap is very thin and has eroded (arrow), allowing contact between the lipid pool and the thrombus.
x18 Picro-Mallory trichrome.

6.29 Coronary thrombosis. In this angiogram the thrombus shown in **6.28** is seen as a filling defect in the column of barium. This appearance is characteristic of large thrombi and is exactly what the clinician can demonstrate by angiography in life.

6.30 Coronary thrombosis. Complete thrombotic occlusion of a coronary artery due to plaque rupture. There is a large intimal plaque encircling most of the artery. This plaque has lost its fibrous cap over a large area, and the defect (arrows) is filled by thrombus which extends deep into the plaque and also occludes the lumen of the artery. Injection medium is also present in the plaque, having tracked from the more proximal vessel where there was a lumen. At the point shown in this section the lumen is totally occluded by thrombus.
x25 Elastic-hematoxylin and eosin.

6.31 Coronary thrombosis. Trichrome-stained section adjacent to that shown in **6.30**. The thrombus in the lumen contains abundant fibrin (red) and red cells (orange), as does the more superficial thrombus in the intima. The deeper thrombus in the intima at the junction with the plaque lipid (arrow) is stained purple, indicating a higher proportion of platelets.
x25 Picro-Mallory trichrome.

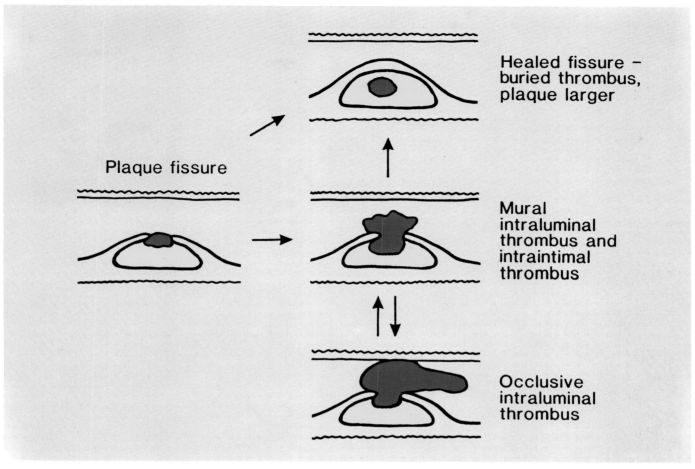

Plaque fissure

Healed fissure – buried thrombus, plaque larger

Mural intraluminal thrombus and intraintimal thrombus

Occlusive intraluminal thrombus

6.32 Evolution of plaque fissures and coronary thrombi

6.32 Evolution of plaque fissures and coronary thrombi. The ability of cardiologists to carry out serial coronary arteriograms on patients with early acute myocardial infarction and crescendo angina, has radically altered concepts concerning coronary thrombi. In these patients, coronary thrombi can be identified as filling defects within the vessel lumen. In the early stages, thrombi are consistently found in the artery supplying an area of infarction. These thrombi may rapidly lyse spontaneously or with the use of thrombolytic therapy, or grow to totally occlude the lumen. These changes take place over a few hours or days. Pathological studies have contributed the fact that virtually all these thrombi are related to plaque fissures. It is, therefore, now possible to construct the sequence of events which follow plaque rupture. Following the initial tear, thrombus develops both within the plaque from blood dissecting into the intima and on the intimal surface over the tear. The intra-intimal component may be very large and cause sudden plaque expansion occluding the lumen. The intraluminal thrombus may also grow to occlude the lumen. Such occlusive thrombi may spontaneously lyse or, particularly if lipid is extruded from the plaque, propagate distally. In the latter case the thrombi usually undergo organization rather than lysis. Healing of plaque fissures involves sealing of the tear with lysis of the mural thrombus. The intra-intimal thrombus usually organizes, having led to a significant increase in plaque growth.

6.33 Experimental myocardial infarction. The left circumflex artery was occluded in a dog for 2 hours after which flow was restored and the animal sacrificed at 12 hours. In the slice of myocardium which has been stained to show succinic dehydrogenase activity there is a recent infarct. The area of infarction is demonstrated as a pale area where enzyme activity has been lost. The infarction is regional in that it involves the lateral wall of the left ventricle only, but it is not transmural and the subpericardial zone is spared.

6.34 Recent myocardial infarction. Transverse slice across the ventricles (short axis view). On the lateral wall of the left ventricle an area of necrosis is visible (arrows) which involves almost the whole thickness of the myocardium. The acute infarction is regional in distribution and from the history it was of 7 days duration. The centre of the infarct is yellow with a red rim where there is vascular proliferation as organization begins.

6.35, 6.36, 6.37 Recent myocardial infarction. Transverse sections across the ventricles from three patients with acute myocardial infarction, which have been stained to demonstrate succinic dehydrogenase activity. Presence of the enzyme in normal muscle is shown by a purple end-product. Dead muscle which has lost enzyme activity remains pale.

In **6.35** there is the typical antero-septal infarct that follows occlusion of the left anterior descending coronary artery. The area of necrosis (pale-staining) involves the anterior wall of the left ventricle and the anterior two-thirds of the septum. A sub-endocardial extension of the main infarct is common. Even in the area of infarction a small rim of surviving blue-staining myocardium is present just beneath the endocardium.

In **6.36** there is the typical posterior infarct that follows occlusion of the right coronary artery. The area of necrosis involves the posterior wall of the left ventricle, the posterior third of the septum, and the right ventricle. On the lateral wall of the left ventricle is a small fibrous scar of a previous infarct.

In **6.37** there is a small regional lateral infarct due to occlusion of the left circumflex artery which also involves the antero-lateral papillary muscle.

6.38 Regional subendocardial infarction. Transverse section across the ventricles stained by succinic dehydrogenase activity. The enzyme loss indicating recent infarction is in the antero-septal region but does not involve the full thickness of the ventricular wall. There is also an old fibrous scar on the posterior wall.

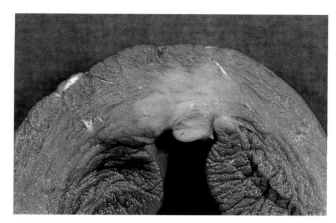
6.33 Experimental myocardial infarction

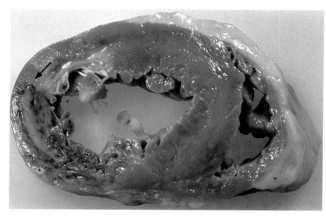
6.34 Recent infarction

6.39 Diffuse subendocardial necrosis. Transverse slice across the ventricles stained for succinic dehydrogenase activity. There is enzyme loss in the inner two-thirds of the whole circumference of the left ventricle. The right ventricle is normally stained. The pattern of necrosis in this case is not regional but diffuse and sub-endocardial. This pattern of necrosis indicates an overall fall in perfusion throughout the myocardium.

6.40 Acute myocardial infarction of mixed type. Transverse slice across the ventricles stained for succinic dehydrogenase activity. Numerous areas of enzyme loss are scattered throughout the left ventricles. In the septum, infarction is virtually full-thickness but elsewhere it takes the form of irregular foci which vary in size from a few millimetres to over 1cm across and are not regional in distribution. The postero-lateral wall of the ventricle shows a dense pearly-white scar of an old healed infarct. The pattern of necrosis in this case is a complex mixture of regional and diffuse types. This pattern is common in the end stage of coronary atheroma where all three main arteries are diffusely narrowed.

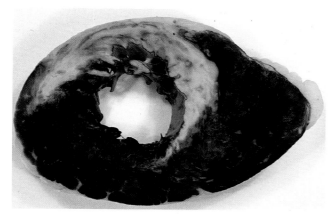

6.35 Recent infarction

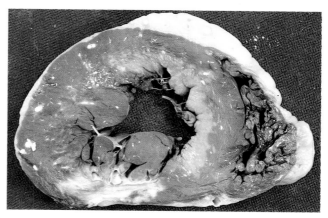

6.38 Regional subendocardial infarction

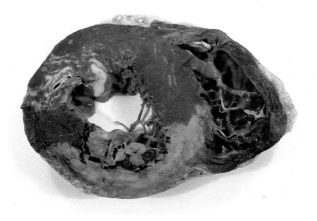

6.36 Recent infarction

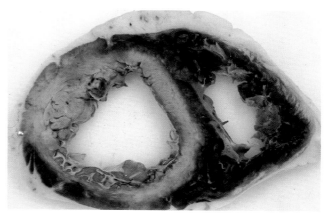

6.39 Diffuse subendocardial necrosis

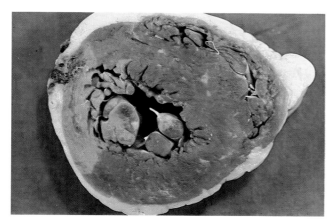

6.37 Recent infarction

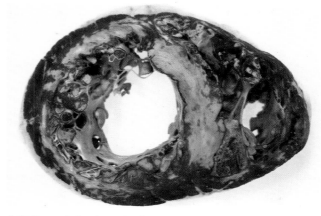

6.40 Recent infarction: mixed type

MORPHOLOGICAL CHANGES
IN ISCHEMIC MYOCARDIAL DAMAGE

Complex classifications and descriptions exist of the myocardial changes occurring in man; in reality most cases contain mixtures of all these types. Guides as to how to assess the duration of ischemic damage are also published, but many human infarcts contain areas which are apparently of different ages.

In animal models of infarction, where the onset of ischemia can be exactly timed, the morphological changes have been described and act as a guide to the significance of similar changes in man.

Even in simple animal models where the occlusion is instantaneous and complete, the infarct shows a spectrum of changes suggesting that infarction is a dynamic and evolving process. The proportion of dead myocardial cells within the ischemic zone rises in a linear relation with time becoming total only after 6 hours' occlusion.

METABOLIC CONSEQUENCES
OF ISCHEMIC MYOCARDIAL DAMAGE

Complete occlusion of a coronary artery in the dog leads to complete cessation of the contractile activity of that segment of myocardium within a minute. Within this short period tissue oxygen levels fall and mitochondrial energy production switches to anaerobic glycolysis as the means by which high energy phosphates are generated. The cessation of contraction reduces the energy demand but, even so, there is a steady fall in the intracellular levels of high energy phosphate. Intracellular breakdown of ATP and ADP associated with lactate accumulation, lead to increasing intracellular acidosis. Anaerobic glycolysis is ultimately unable to generate enough energy to maintain membrane integrity, largely because the glycogen stores are finite and accumulating lactate inhibits key enzyme reactions. Once membrane function is impaired K^+ ions leave the cell and Na^+ and water pour in. Ca^{++} ions also enter the cell and the mitochondria. The exact point at which the cell suffers irreversible damage is not entirely certain but once Ca^{++} ions have accumulated within mitochondria and intracellular enzymes are being lost to the extracellular space, the damage is irreversible.

STRUCTURAL CHANGES
DUE TO ISCHEMIC DAMAGE
IN EXPERIMENTAL REGIONAL INFARCTION

Electron microscopy will detect changes such as glycogen depletion and mitochondrial swelling within 40 minutes of arterial occlusion. Changes detectable by light microscopy are not evident for 6-8 hours after which they become steadily more recognizable.

Infiltration of the area by polymorphs begins early and may be seen before the hypereosinophilia and loss of myofibrillary cross striations makes the death of the myocardial cell apparent. Polymorphs increase in numbers up to three days and thereafter remain only as degenerate pyknotic forms. Macrophages appear at four to five days. Regional infarction involves large areas in which both the myocardial cells and the stromal tissue have been destroyed. This necrosis of the microvasculature ensures that the centre of the infarct is avascular and that an inflammatory response cannot develop. In this central area the muscle cells become hyaline and amorphous and the nuclei vanish. Repair of an area of infarction in which the stroma has been destroyed takes place by invasion of the area by new capillaries and fibroblasts growing in from the viable tissue at the margins. In this marginal zone the myocardial cells have often been lost but the stroma remains to form a broad zone of granulation tissue round the infarct, by 7 to 10 days. The invasion of the amorphous dead muscle by capillaries and fibroblasts is stimulated by release of a myocardial angiogenesis factor structurally very similar to tumour angiogenesis factor. Complete collagenous replacement takes up to six months.

In experimental animals it is possible to re-establish flow at an interval of time short of that required to produce necrosis of every myocardial cell. Under these circumstances somewhat different morphological changes occur. The myocardial cell is subjected to a massive influx of Ca^{++} ions and water from the plasma reperfusing the interstitial tissues. The calcium accumulates within the mitochondria as crystalline deposits and invokes intense supercontraction of the myofibrils. This 'rigor' shortens the cell, often leading to mechanical disruption of the cell membrane. The contracted sarcomas are visible by light microscopy as bright eosinophilic cross bands within the cell. The appearances are so striking that they can be recognized far earlier than the 'coagulation' of myofibrils that occurs in non-reperfused infarcted muscle.

MORPHOLOGICAL CHANGES FOLLOWING ISCHEMIA IN MAN (6.41 – 6.54)

Large areas of regional infarction, particularly those which are transmural, develop 'coagulative' necrosis in which both myocardial cells and the stroma die. The sequence of changes which converts such infarcts to fibrous scars is identical to that described in the dog myocardium.

Contraction band necrosis is also common in man and it is logical to assume that this represents ischemic damage followed by reperfusion. Identical changes occur in damaged myocardial cells from many causes, for example at the margins of cardiac biopsies.

In man microscopic focal areas of necrosis are found in which the stromal cells survive and the myocardial cell cytoplasm is rapidly removed by macrophages, following which the stroma collapses to leave a focal scar containing residual lipofuscin. Fibroblastic proliferation within areas which have stromal survival is very rapid and florid. This form of necrosis may occur as focal areas at the margins of larger areas of complete infarction, or may occur independently in foci which range widely in size. The microscopic focal form is predominantly found in the subendocardial zone, but similar foci occur in the subpericardial zone when microemboli have occurred.

In man a further expression of ischemic damage is what is known as myocytolysis. The myocardial cells are large and vacuolated to a degree at which myofibrillary structure is virtually lost. The change is thought to reflect cells which are viable but have lost the ability to maintain normal fluid balance and to synthesize myofibrillary protein. Lesser degrees of the change are seen in which the cells are swollen and 'moth-eaten' in appearance but still contain recognized myofibrils. Myocytolysis is often seen in the myocardial cells immediately beneath the endocardium and in the papillary muscles in patients with ischemic myocardial necrosis.

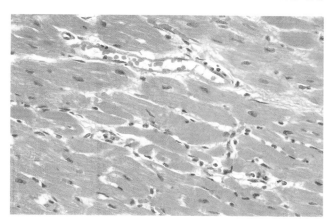

6.41 Early infarction

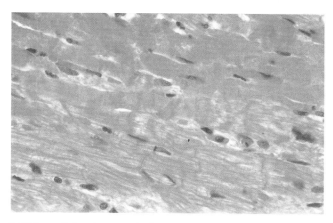

6.42 Acute infarction: marginal zone

6.41 Early acute myocardial infarction: histology. Myocardium in which there is a small focus of hypereosinophilic muscle fibres, some of which show 'contraction' bands. These are hypereosinophilic dense cross bands in the cytoplasma; they represent areas of hypertonic contraction which shunt myofibrils together. There are a few interstitial inflammatory cells, but the stromal tissues appear viable and the surrounding myocardial fibres are normal.
x225 Hematoxylin and eosin.

6.42 Acute myocardial infarction: marginal zone. An area of acute myocardial infarction. Two groups of myocardial cells are present, one shows hypereosinophilia and contraction bands. The other group shows slight swelling and vacuolation. The former are undoubtedly dead, the latter may recover.
x275 Hematoxylin and eosin.

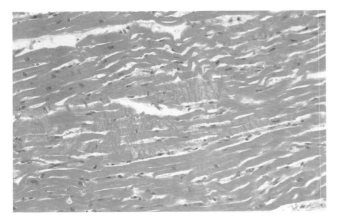

6.43 Early infarction

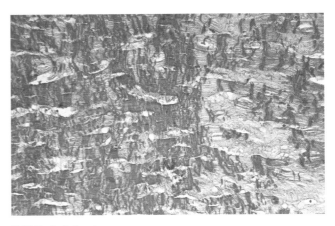

6.44 Early infarction

6.43 Early acute myocardial infarction: histology.
Focal area of myocardial fibres which show contraction
bands as an indication of ischemic damage. This is the
earliest morpholigical indication of ischemic damage to
the myocardium although it is not entirely specific. It
represents shunting together or hypercontraction of some
myofibrils in the cells as a form of intracellular rigor.
x175 Hematoxylin and eosin.

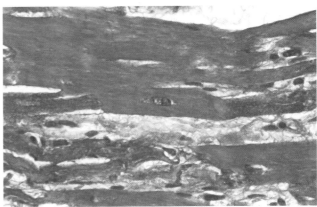

6.45 Early infarction

6.44 Early acute myocardial infarction: histology.
Contraction bands can be made more easily identifiable
by all the numerous technical variations on acid and basic
fuchsin stains. The hypercontracted segments retain the
fuchsin stain, appearing bright red.
x175 Acid fuchsin.

6.45 Early acute myocardial infarction. A focal area
of ischemic myocardial necrosis. The section is stained by
the Picro-Mallory technique in which muscle fibres stain
red. Immediately adjacent to these normal cells are dead
muscle cells, some actually abutting onto viable cells. The
dead myocardial cells are shrunken and have lost the
myofibrillary staining, appearing blue. This intimate
mixture of dead and living muscle cells is typical of the
marginal zones of acute infarction.
x375 Picro-Mallory trichrome.

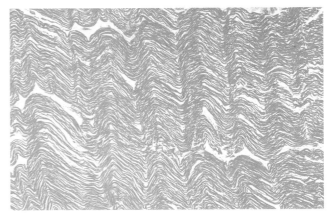

6.46 Early infarction

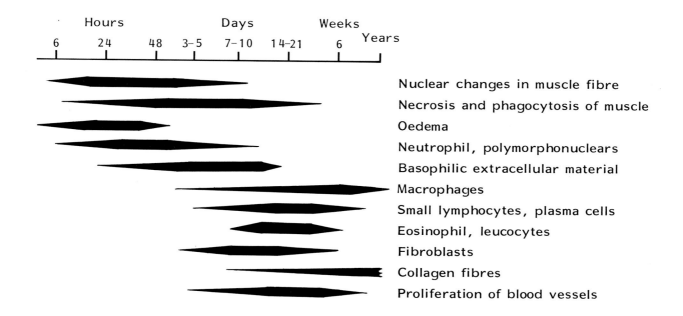

6.47 Dating of myocardial infarction

6.46 Early acute myocardial infarction. Wavy fibres as an indication of myocardial infarction. The muscle fibres are thrown into regular folds. This appearance is best seen in a patient who has a large infarct and survives some hours with good contraction in the adjacent areas of myocardium. The appearance is of little practical help in recognizing infarction at an early stage.
x40 Hematoxylin and eosin.

6.47 Diagrammatic representation of dating of histological appearances in acute myocardial infarction. This scheme is the best that can be done to attempt to determine the age of an area of myocardial infarction in man from its histological appearance. The difficulty in this exercise is that the changes do not progress evenly over the whole area of infarction. In assessing the age, the marginal areas of infarction are probably the most reliable. This approach can be criticized, however, because there is good clinical evidence that infarcts may increase in size over some days. On the other hand, the central area of an infarct may retain necrotic hyaline muscle for many months although the margins are mature collagen. *(Diagram reproduced by courtesy of Dr. I.C. Lodge-Patch.)*

6.48   Focal myocardial necrosis. There is a focal area in which the cytoplasm of the myocardial cells has vanished, leaving open spaces in the interstitial tissue which has survived. Lipofuscin derived from dead muscle cells is present in macrophages in the area.
x250 Hematoxylin and eosin.

6.49   Focal ischemic scarring. Focal area of fibrous scarring resulting from the healing of the process shown in **6.48**. Such scars, while most commonly due to ischemia, can be caused by other factors, because they are also found in ventricular hypertrophy, metabolic disorders and all cardiomyopathies.
x200 Hematoxylin and eosin.

6.50   Acute infarction: myocytolysis. Acute myocardial infarction in which the majority of cells are hyper-eosinophilic and have lost their nuclei. The central focus of muscle cells around a small blood vessel is vacuolated with loss of myofibrils but apparently viable nuclei remain. Electron microscopy can show that such cells have large empty spaces, but mitochondria are present and still contain demonstrable enzyme activity. The potential of these cells to return to normal is uncertain.
x225 Hematoxylin and eosin.

6.51   Acute myocardial infarction at 4 days. Acute myocardial infarction showing the acute inflammatory response at the margin of the area of dead muscle. The myocardial fibres are totally amorphous and lack nuclei. Towards one edge there is an interstitial infiltrate of polymorphonuclear leukocytes between the dead cells. This zone of polymorph infiltration does not reach the centre of the infarct.
x200 Hematoxylin and eosin.

6.52   Acute myocardial infarction at 7-10 days. Acute myocardial infarction with a central focus of eosinophilic necrotic myocardial cells around which there is a zone of florid granulation tissue containing macrophages, proliferating fibroblasts and new blood vessels. This organization of the area of necrosis begins at approximately 5-7 days and continues until the infarct is replaced by collagen. No regeneration of cardiac muscle occurs.
x175 Hematoxylin and eosin.

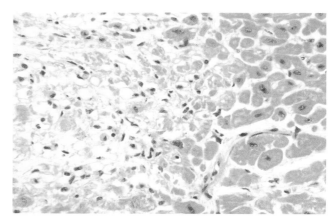

6.48 Focal myocardial necrosis

6.53   Acute myocardial infarction: organization phase. Vascular granulation tissue is shown at the margin of a large area of eosinophilic necrotic myocardial cells. The histiocytic response has largely disappeared.
x150 Hematoxylin and eosin.

6.54   Acute myocardial infarction: healing phase. A focus of myocardial cells has been replaced by granulation tissue which still contains a number of chronic inflammatory cells. At the margin of the area of muscle loss, one surviving fibre has developed enlarged and hyperchromatic nuclei. The muscle cells at the margin of scars become polyploid; this is the closest that the cardiac muscle comes to developing regenerative giant cells in the manner seen in skeletal muscle.
x175 Hematoxylin and eosin.

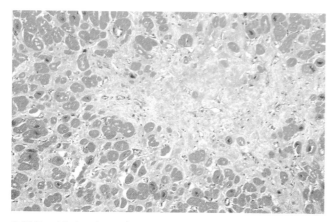

6.49 Focal ischemic scarring

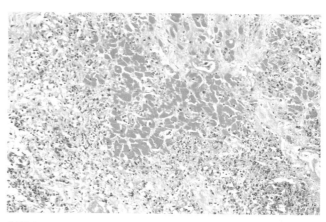

6.52 Acute infarction: 7–10 days

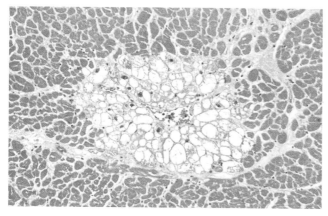

6.50 Acute infarction: myocytolysis

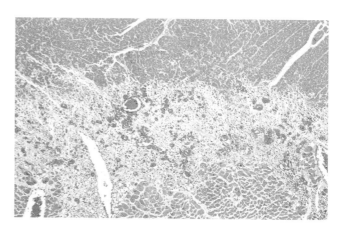

6.53 Acute infarction: organization phase

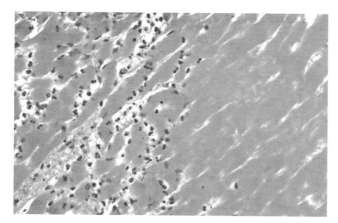

6.51 Acute infarction: 4 days

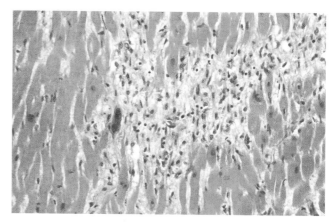

6.54 Acute infarction: healing phase

SEQUELAE OF MYOCARDIAL INFARCTION (6.55 – 6.67)

The most significant result of acute regional myocardial infarction is death from the sudden onset of ventricular fibrillation. This complication, usually occurring within the first 24 hours after onset of chest pain, is not directly related to the size of the infarct. In contrast, cardiogenic shock and acute left ventricular failure steadily increase in incidence when larger areas of necrosis are present.

In the acute phase of acute myocardial infarction, around 5% of the mortality is due to cardiac rupture leading to hemopericardium. Rupture is caused both by excavation of soft yellow infarcts at about the 5 to 7 day period and by a tear between the area of necrosis and the normal myocardium in infarcts of much shorter duration. Internal rupture leads to the creation of an acute ventricular septal defect and a sudden left-to-right shunt. Myocardial rupture is a complication solely of transmural infarction. Rupture of a papillary muscle may involve one small sub-head, or a major portion leading to sudden torrential regurgitation. The infarction leading to these papillary muscle ruptures is often small and not necessarily transmural.

In approximately one-third of fatal cases of acute myocardial infarction, the endocardial surface of the area of necrosis is covered by ante-mortem thrombus acting as a potential source of systemic emboli.

In the resolution of an acute myocardial infarct, the necrotic muscle is ultimately replaced by fibrous tissue. The scars of such healed infarcts are clearly visible in post-mortem hearts. When infarction was transmural, the resulting fibrous tissue may develop an aneurysmal bulge some weeks after the acute episode. These aneurysms frequently contain mural thrombus. The clinical sequelae are those of cardiac failure and systemic emboli. Actual rupture of aneurysms is rare but may occur. Widespread ischemic damage may produce very diffuse fibrosis with an evenly dilated thin-walled left ventricle. There is a complete spectrum from localized saccular to very diffuse aneurysms, all of which may or may not contain thrombus. A rarer acute ventricular aneurysm results from expansion of large transmural infarcts due to tearing and sliding of muscle bundles within the necrotic tissue and usually ends as myocardial rupture.

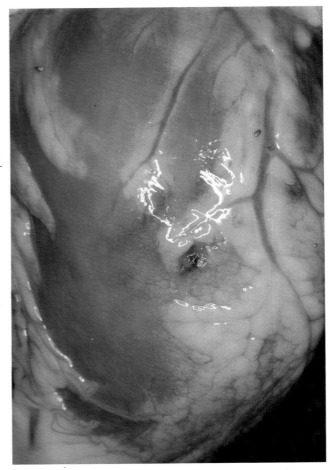

6.55 Acute infarction: external rupture

6.55 Acute myocardial infarction: external rupture. A small slit-like tear is present on the pericardial surface of an acute posterior myocardial infarction. The patient died of a hemopericardium on the second day after onset of chest pain. The ventricular rupture ranges from small slits to large ragged tears.

References:

Feneley M P, Chang V P and O'Rouke M F. Myocardial rupture after acute myocardial infarction. Ten year review. Br Heart J 1983; 49: 550-556.

Svendsen F and Harveit F. Cardiac rupture over 2 decades before and after the introduction of external cardiac compression. International Journal of Cardiology 1984; 5: 530-531.

Vlodaver Z and Edwards J E. Rupture of ventricular septum or papillary muscle complicating myocardial infarction. Circulation 1977; 55: 815-822.

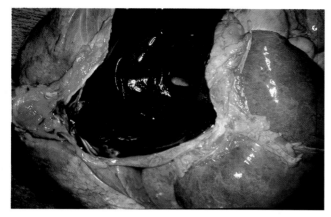

6.56 Hemopericardium

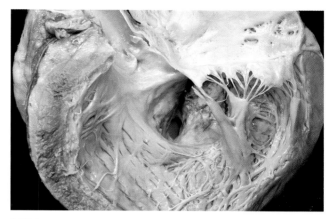

6.58 Acute infarction: internal rupture

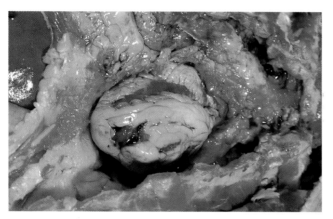

6.57 Hemopericardium

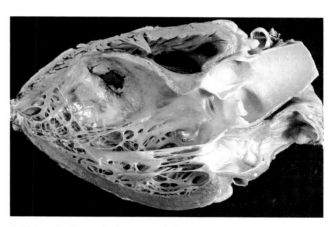

6.59 Acquired ventricular septal defect

6.56 Hemopericardium due to external cardiac rupture. The pericardial sac has been opened to show that it contains over a litre of blood clot which was under some pressure. A leak this large always indicates a significant lesion. Where there is a tear in the left ventricle of a patient in whom external massage has been enthusiastically carried out, and only 200-300mls of blood present in the pericardium, it is difficult to decide whether the finding is the cause of death. It may merely be an agonal event produced by resuscitation.

6.57 Hemopericardium due to external cardiac rupture. The same case as **6.56** is illustrated after removal of the blood clot from the pericardium. There is a 3cm split in the anterior wall of the left ventricle through a recent infarct. Clinical history of 3 hours only. While often regarded as a complication developing on day 5-7, cardiac rupture is equally common in very early infarction.

6.58 Acute myocardial infarction: internal rupture. The left ventricle has been opened to show the left side of the interventricular septum. Posteriorly just behind the postero-medial papillary muscle is an aneurysmal bulge with an oval hole which communicates with the right ventricle. The patient developed a left-to-right shunt soon after an acute posterior myocardial infarct and survived for two months.

6.59 Acquired ventricular septal defect. A long axis view of the left ventricle is shown. A diffuse anteroseptal aneurysm has ruptured through the anterior portion of the septum into the right ventricle.

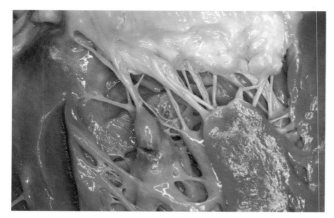

6.60 Acute infarction: papillary muscle rupture

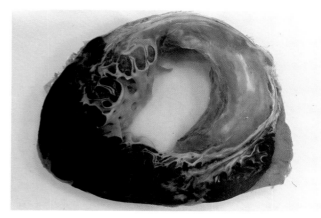

6.62 Ventricular aneurysm with thrombosis

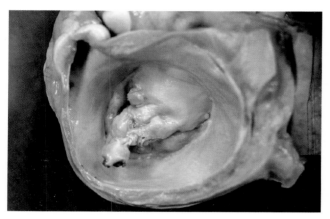

6.61 Acute infarction: papillary muscle rupture

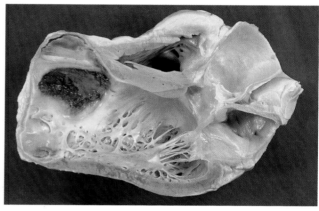

6.63 Ischemic aneurysm

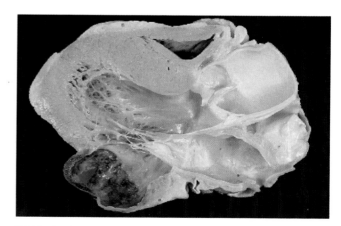

6.64 Ischemic aneurysm

6.60 Acute myocardial infarction: papillary muscle rupture. Mitral valve opened to show partial avulsion of the posterior medial papillary muscle in a patient with acute myocardial infarction. The papillary muscle stump was still attached to the ventricular wall and had not prolapsed into the atrium.

6.61 Acute myocardial infarction: papillary muscle rupture. Left atrium opened to show the mitral valve from above, in a patient who died with torrential mitral regurgitation following an acute myocardial infarction. The stump of a ruptured papillary muscle tangled in chordae is present in the atrium. The stump of the papillary muscle had been constantly passing between the atria and ventricle in a flail-like motion.

6.62 Left ventricular aneurysm with thrombosis. Transverse section through the ventricles in a patient who died some months after an acute regional anterior myocardial infarction. The myocardium is coloured dark blue following staining to demonstrate succinic dehydrogenase activity. The anterior wall of the left ventricle is composed of thin fibrous tissue which has bulged outward as an aneurysmal sac filled with laminated red thrombus.

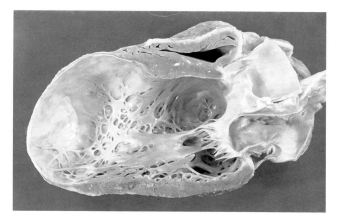

6.65 Ischemic apical aneurysm

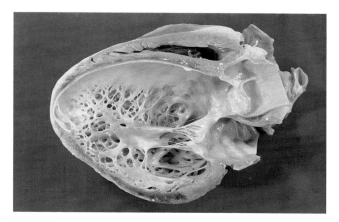

6.66 Diffuse apical ischemic aneurysm

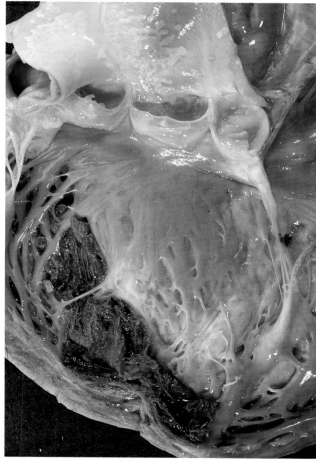

6.67 Ischemic aneurysmal dilation

6.63   Ischemic aneurysm of left ventricle. Long-axis plane through a heart in which there is an apical aneurysm containing mural thrombus. Thrombus has virtually filled and sealed the aneurysm sac.

6.64   Ischemic aneurysm of left ventricle. Long-axis plane through a heart in which there is a posterior ischemic aneurysm behind the papillary muscle in the left ventricle. The aneurysm is thin-walled and ruptured to cause death five months after the acute infarction. This aneurysm has a thin wall and was constantly filled with blood since it did not develop a large amount of thrombus. The aneurysm is well defined, the immediately adjacent myocardium is normal.

6.65   Ischemic apical aneurysm of left ventricle. Long axis view of the left ventricle. This aneurysm is confined to the apical trabeculated portion of the ventricle which is symmetrically dilated. The aneurysm is thin-

walled with marked endocardial thickening but no mural thrombus. It filled paradoxically in systole.

6.66   Diffuse apical ischemic aneurysm of left ventricle. Long axis view of the left ventricle. In contrast to **6.65** this aneurysm involves virtually the whole left ventricle, whose diameter is greatly increased. There is diffuse endocardial thickening shown by a white opaque appearance, but thrombus is absent in this case.

6.67   Ischemic aneurysmal dilation of left ventricle. A dilated thin-walled ventricle due to severe stenosis of all three coronary arteries and diffuse myocardial fibrosis. The cavity is dilated and mural thrombus has developed over much of the anterior wall and septum. The patient did not have any chest pain, presenting with arrhythmias and cardiac failure; the misleading term 'ischemic cardiomyopathy' is sometimes used by clinicians for this condition.

CHAPTER 7

Cardiomyopathy and Myocarditis

No universally accepted and logical usage of the terms cardiomyopathy and myocarditis has yet been evolved. There is general agreement that these terms cover myocardial diseases which are not due to interference with the coronary blood flow (ischemic), nor secondary to the effects of volume or pressure overload on the myocardium from valvar disease or congenital shunts.

In the most recent terminology proposed by the World Health Organization it is suggested that the term cardiomyopathy be limited to heart muscle disease of unknown cause: a definition close to what others have called primary cardiomyopathy. The term specific heart muscle disease is used by the WHO when there is a known cause or associated systemic disease, i.e. close to what has been known as secondary cardiomyopathy.

The term myocarditis is also used widely in both clinical and pathological fields without a precise definition. In the former it invokes an impression of the rapid onset of cardiac symptoms with fever, in the latter the finding of inflammatory cells in the myocardium. While the latter is more specific, it does involve a cardiac biopsy or autopsy for its usage; moreover, some viral infections of the myocardium always called 'myocarditis' are characterized by necrosis with a minimal inflammatory response.

DILATED CARDIOMYOPATHY (7.1 – 7.7)

Within the group of diseases known as cardiomyopathies, as defined above, a functional classification based on left ventricular contraction is widely used clinically, and it does have some morphological correlates at macroscopic level.

In terms of function, congestive or dilated cardiomyopathy has poor systolic contraction caused by a diffuse myocardial abnormality. The increase in ventricular muscle mass is the main indicator of cardiac hypertrophy, but the striking feature is the dilatation of the ventricular cavities with a reduced wall thickness. In many patients coming to autopsy, mural thrombus has developed in the crevices of either ventricle and in the atrial appendages.

At a histological level, the striking feature of dilated cardiomyopathy is an increase in interstitial fibrosis. This follows a continuing cycle of loss of muscle fibres, a process that recalls piecemeal necrosis of the liver progressing to cirrhosis. Tiny foci of individual cell necrosis to which a localized inflammatory response has occurred can be found to a variable degree in all cases. Cases in which this is a prominent feature are sometimes labelled 'myocarditis'.

The histological features are non-specific and do not in themselves point to any particular etiology. It is likely that the dilated form of cardiomyopathy is the end-stage of diffuse myocardial damage from many causes. An association between some cases of dilated cardiomyopathy and previous acute viral myocarditis, either overt or subclinical, has been suggested. High titres to Coxsackie virus have been shown in a limited number of clinical cases with short histories. It is proposed that acute viral myocarditis is in most cases a self-limiting disease with either complete recovery or death, in the acute phase, from massive myocardial involvement. A tiny proportion of cases apparently recover and pass into a 'cardiomyopathy' after a latent period. Cases of dilated cardiomyopathy without an acute history may have had subclinical viral infection. While virus infection is likely to be the cause in some instances, an exactly similar end-stage morphological picture is found in alcohol abuse as well as in cobalt-induced myocardial damage; other cases are familial with or without an associated skeletal myopathy. It is thus clear that a congestive cardiomyopathy is the end-stage of myocardial damage from many causes and, if the cause is not apparent clinically, histological examination of the myocardium is unlikely to be more rewarding.

HYPERTROPHIC CARDIOMYOPATHY (7.8 – 7.14)

In this entity, systolic function is hyperkinetic and virtually obliterates the ventricular cavity, producing in some cases an apparent obstruction to the outflow. All cases show a reduced systolic volume and marked difficulty in diastolic filling. The question of whether real obstruction to outflow exists is debated by clinicians. It is undoubtedly true that a pressure gradient exists across the ventricular outflow, but by this phase of contraction the ventricle has already largely emptied.

The original morphological descriptions by Teare, of hypertrophic cardiomyopathy, were concentrated on cases with asymmetrical thickening of the ventricular septum. It has since been realized by both clinicians and pathologists that the disease can occur in many other forms. It may involve left, right or both ventricles, and within either ventricle it can be symmetrical or asymmetrical. If asymmetrical, the area of abnormal myocardium may be at any site and is not always septal. The disease can even be found in hearts of normal size which macroscopically show no abnormalities. Thus hypertrophic cardiomyopathy can occur in hearts which are not hypertrophic, using the criterion of an increase in muscle mass. None of the other cardiomyopathies are as protean in their manifestation at a macroscopic level. In hypertrophic cardiomyopathy a highly characteristic forward movement of the anterior cusp of the mitral valve toward the septum occurs in systole (SAM), obliterating the left ventricular outflow. The mitral valve cusp hits the ventricular septum with considerable force and leads to a diagnostic patch of endocardial thickening just below the aortic valve.

Histologically, hypertrophic cardiomyopathy has what is close to a specific morphology. Within the areas of affected myocardium there is considerable interstitial fibrosis with a striking mal-arrangement or whorling of the muscle fibres. Within the myocardial cell at ultrastructural level, myofibrillary disarray is present. The cell-to-cell orientation of muscle cells is lost, leading to the circular whorls of myocardial fibres. When present to any degree, these changes are diagnostic but are not totally specific. In normal hearts some mal-arrangement, but without the other histological abnormalities, is found at the junction of the septum with the anterior and posterior walls of the left ventricle. Congenitally abnormal hearts may also show fibre disarray. The whole question of absolute specificity has recently been a matter of controversy, but given the whole heart at autopsy the diagnosis is not usually difficult. The condition cannot, however, be diagnosed or excluded from examination of a single histological section or biopsy.

As regards etiology, hypertrophic cardiomyopathy is a more homogeneous entity than dilated cardiomyopathy and is probably always familial. Accumulating evidence suggests that the myocardium has an abnormal sensitivity to catecholamines, leading to alterations is the myocardial fibre shape which perhaps dates from before birth. The disease is in some cases associated with disorders of neural crest tissue including neurofibromatosis, lentiginosis and pheochromocytoma. In Friedreich's ataxia, the heart is also very like hypertrophic cardiomyopathy at a functional and histological level, but it seldom develops the full macroscopic picture.

RESTRICTIVE AND OBLITERATIVE CARDIOMYOPATHY (7.15 – 7.20)

In pure restrictive cardiomyopathy the endocardium or myocardium is abnormally stiff, resulting in the ventricles filling in diastole only at high pressures. Systolic contractile function and cavity size are normal. In this pure form, the cause may be deposition of amyloid on the basement membrane of myocardial cells or the early stages of endomyocardial fibrosis (EMF). In the later phase of endomyocardial fibrosis, steady obliteration of the cavities of the ventricles occurs, starting at the apex. This process spreads, involving the atrioventricular valves and leading to regurgitation but sparing the outflow tracts and aortic and pulmonary valves. Finally, severe reduction in ventricular systolic contraction occurs. In the early acute phase of the disease, thrombotic material is deposited on the endocardial surface; it is largely the organization of this deposit that leads to the dense fibrosis which obliterates the ventricular cavity. The fibrosis fuses the trabeculae and papillary muscles of the ventricle into a solid mass. Evidence has now emerged to show that the non-tropical form of EMF is related to a circulating eosinophilia; degranulation of such cells produces a factor which damages the endocardium. Tropical EMF is not yet proven to be constantly related to previous or present eosinophilia but is otherwise identical in morphological appearances to that found in non-tropical countries.

References:

Brigden W. Uncommon myocardial diseases. The non-coronary cardiomyopathies. Lancet 1957; 2: 1179-1184.

Davies M J. Invited review. The cardiomyopathies: a review of terminology, pathology and pathogenesis. Histopathology 1984; 8: 363-394.

Goodwin J F. The frontiers of cardiomyopathy. Br Heart J 1982; 48: 1-18.

Just H and Schuster H P eds. Myocarditis and Cardiomyopathy. Berlin: Springer 1983.

Perloff J K. Pathogenesis of hypertrophic cardiomyopathy – hypothesis and speculation. Am Heart J 1981; 101: 219-226.

World Health Organization. Report of the WHO/ISFC task force on the definition and classification of cardiomyopathies. Br Heart J 1980; 44: 672-673.

7.1 Dilated cardiomyopathy. Macroscopic specimen of the heart from a child dying of congestive cardiomyopathy. Other members of the family had a similar disease. The heart is enlarged and globular with a dilated left ventricle whose cavity diameter is increased but the wall thickness is within normal limits. Mural thrombus is present on left ventricular endocardium.

7.2 Dilated cardiomyopathy. The left ventricle has been opened to show the aortic valve and interventricular septum in an adult patient dying of idiopathic congestive cardiomyopathy. Mural thrombus is present between and beneath the trabeculae of the left ventricular myocardium. The ventricle is dilated and globular in shape.

7.3 Dilated cardiomyopathy. Histological section of left ventricular muscle in a man of 38 with idiopathic congestive cardiomyopathy. The majority of myocardial fibres are seen in cross-section. There is marked variation in muscle fibre diameter, and interstitial fibrosis separates individual myocardial cells. Many of the myocardial cells appear vacuolated, the vacuoles appearing empty or containing slightly basophilic amorphous material.
x550 Hematoxylin and eosin.

7.4 Dilated cardiomyopathy. Trichrome-stained section of a left ventricular biopsy in idiopathic congestive cardiomyopathy. The purple-stained myocardial fibres vary in diameter and are separated by blue-staining collagen in the interstitial tissue.
x325 Mallory trichrome stain.

7.5 Dilated cardiomyopathy. Van Gieson-stained histological section of the myocardium at post-mortem in congestive cardiomyopathy. The brown-staining muscle fibres are embedded in a background of red-staining collagen which is present in vast excess as compared to a normal heart.
x100 Van Gieson.

7.6 Dilated cardiomyopathy. Trichrome-stained histological section of left ventricular myocardium in longitudinal plane from a patient with idiopathic congestive cardiomyopathy. The majority of the myocardial fibres are entirely normal and only show some variation in diameter. One fibre has collapsed, being recognizable as deeply basophilic cytoplasmic debris around which the stroma is condensing. Such individual myocardial fibre death can be found to some degree in most cases of idiopathic congestive cardiomyopathy.
x275 Mallory trichrome stain.

7.7 Dilated cardiomyopathy. Section of the left ventricular myocardium in a case of congestive cardiomyopathy associated with high alcohol intake. Relatively

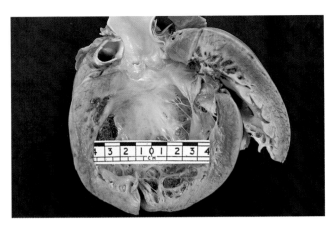

7.1 Dilated cardiomyopathy

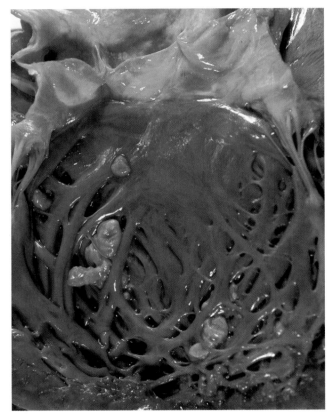

7.2 Dilated cardiomyopathy

normal myocardium abuts onto an area of dense fibrosis within which are embedded isolated myocardial fibres. At the junction between the two zones there are spaces representing empty sarcolemmal tubes within which are macrophages. The appearances represent active muscle fibre loss and are sometimes interpreted as a 'myocarditis'. The process has analogies to piecemeal necrosis of hepatocytes in liver disease.
x275 Hematoxylin and eosin.

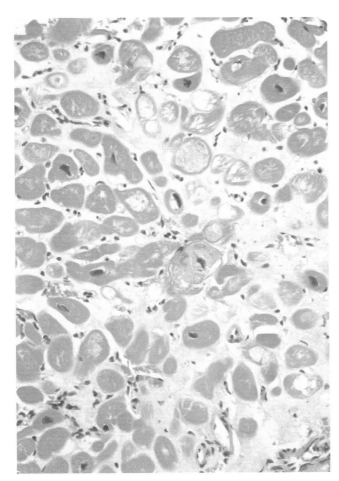

7.3 Dilated cardiomyopathy

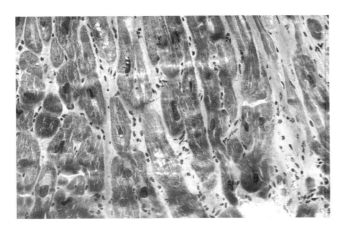

7.4 Dilated cardiomyopathy

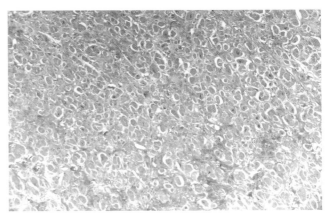

7.5 Dilated cardiomyopathy

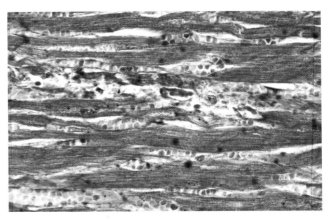

7.6 Dilated cardiomyopathy

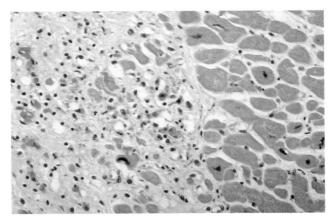

7.7 Dilated cardiomyopathy

7.8 Hypertrophic cardiomyopathy. Hypertrophic cardiomyopathy in a heart opened through the left ventricular outflow and aortic valve, comparable with a long axis view. The muscular interventricular septum bulges across below the aortic valve (A) toward the anterior cusp of the mitral valve (M), narrowing the ventricular outflow. The muscle of the left ventricular wall is thick, with a whorled cut surface resembling that of a uterine fibroid. While opening the heart in this way demonstrates the sub-aortic stenosis, it rather masks recognition of the asymmetry of the ventricle and leads to cases of hypertrophic cardiomyopathy being underdiagnosed by the pathologist.

7.9 Hypertrophic cardiomyopathy. Hypertrophic cardiomyopathy shown in a transverse section across both ventricles at the level of the apices of the papillary muscles. This plane shows the right ventricular outflow (RVO) coming across the anterior surface of the heart. The measurement of the ventricular septum (S) anteriorly is almost 3 times the thickness of the posterior wall (P) of the left ventricle. The case is thus the classic asymmetrical form of hypertrophic cardiomyopathy; but instead of bulging into the left ventricular outflow there is bulging into the right side, producing right ventricular outflow obstruction. This occurs in a small proportion of cases, and hypertrophic cardiomyopathy may produce obstruction of either, both, or neither ventricle. Initially, both clinical and pathological studies were guilty of highlighting only the cases with left-sided obstruction. Transverse sections of the ventricles are the most sensitive method of recognizing hypertrophic cardiomyopathy at autopsy. The cut surface of the septum shows the characteristic 'fibroid-like' appearance of hypertrophic cardiomyopathy.

7.10 Hypertrophic cardiomyopathy. Hypertrophic cardiomyopathy shown in a transverse section across the ventricles. In this case the left ventricular cavity is small, being almost obliterated, and the ventricle is symmetrically thickened with diffuse areas of paler fibrosis throughout the myocardium. The ratio of the septum to posterior wall thickness, while being above the normal limit of 1.4, is only marginally raised and the ventricle is not strikingly asymmetrical. Symmetrical hypertrophy usually occurs when the abnormal muscle is distributed throughout the wide ventricle.

7.11 Hypertrophic cardiomyopathy. Hypertrophic cardiomyopathy with unequivocal clinical and family history but at autopsy a normal heart weight, no left ventricular hypertrophy and a normal cavity size and wall thickness. The only macroscopic abnormality is an unusually thick right ventricle, with a small cavity and large papillary muscles. Histological abnormality was present throughout both ventricles.

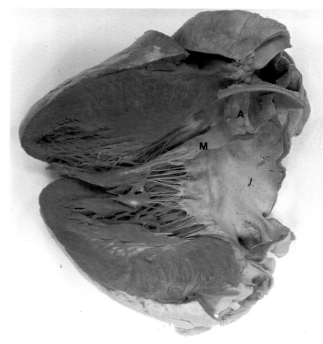

7.8 Hypertrophic cardiomyopathy

7.12 Subaortic endocardial fibrosis in hypertrophic cardiomyopathy. The left ventricular outflow has been opened through the aortic valve in a case of hypertrophic cardiomyopathy. On the interventricular septum below the aortic valve is a transverse band of endocardial thickening with a very sharply-defined lower edge (arrows) exactly at the same level as the lower edge of the anterior cusp of the mitral valve (MV). This feature allows the pathologist to recognize that systolic anterior motion of the anterior cusp had occurred in life. The endocardial thickening is the direct result of impact with the valve cusp; considerable thickening and even destruction of the valve cusp can occur in long-standing cases.

7.13 Hypertrophic cardiomyopathy. Histological section of the left ventricular myocardium in a case of hypertrophic cardiomyopathy. The myocardial fibres are irregular in size, and in the field shown they appear to radiate out from a central focus and then form whorls around foci of loose connective tissue. The nuclei of the myocardial fibres are large and hyperchromatic. x325 Hematoxylin and eosin.

7.14 Hypertrophic cardiomyopathy. A higher-power view from **7.13**. The myocardial fibres are short, broad and irregular in shape. The muscle nuclei are very large. The myofibrillary arrangement within the cells is abnormal, lacking orientation. The myocardial fibres are interspersed with loose connective tissue which contains scattered chronic inflammatory cells. The foci of loose fibrosis contains numerous ovoid nuclei presumably those of fibroblasts.　　　　x375 Hematoxylin and eosin.

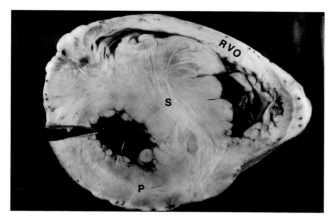

7.9 Hypertrophic cardiomyopathy

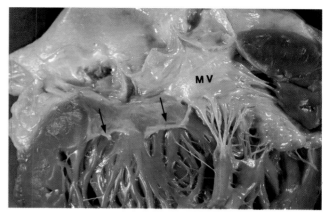

7.12 Subaortic endocardial fibrosis

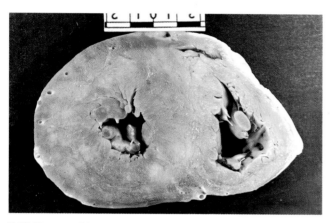

7.10 Hypertrophic cardiomyopathy

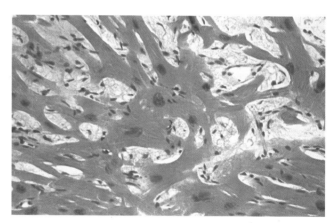

7.13 Hypertrophic cardiomyopathy

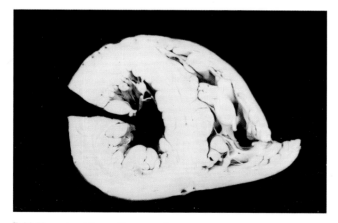

7.11 Hypertrophic cardiomyopathy

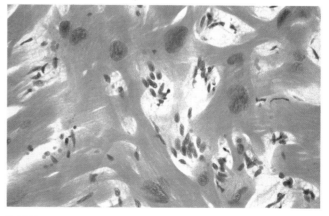

7.14 Hypertrophic cardiomyopathy

References:

Becker A E and Caruso G. Myocardial disarray. A critical review. Br Heart J 1982; 104: 155-155.

Davies M J. The current status of myocardial disarray in hypertrophic cardiomyopathy. Br Heart J 1984; 51: 361-364.

Maron B J and Roberts W C. Hypertrophic cardiomyopathy and cardiac muscle cell disorganisation revisited – relation between the two and significance. Am Heart J 1981; 102: 95-110.

7.15 Endomyocardial fibrosis. Liver biopsy from a man who developed a skin rash with fever and who had a very high blood eosinophilia of unknown cause. The portal tract is densely infiltrated by eosinophils. The patient subsequently died of systemic emboli from endocardial thrombus which was present in both left and right ventricles.
x125 Hematoxylin and eosin.

7.16 Endomyocardial fibrosis. Endocardial thrombus appearing as a flat shaggy coat over the inflow portions of the right ventricle from the case shown in **7.15,** who died in the acute phase of eosinophil-related endomyocardial fibrosis.

7.17 Endomyocardial fibrosis. Section through the thrombus in case shown in **7.15** and **7.16.** The underlying myocardium is normal and does not show fibrous scarring. Superficial to the endocardium are zones of fibrous and granulation tissue containing a number of chronic inflammatory cells but only a very occasional eosinophil. External to these is a zone of recent thrombus. The very regular stratification of these zones is typical.
x40 Hematoxylin and eosin.

7.18 Endomyocardial fibrosis. Trichrome-stained section to show the highly characteristic ordered structure of the endocardial thickening in endomyocardial fibrosis. The myocardium is normal; a discrete zone of vascular blue-staining connective tissue covers the endocardium; and finally there is an external layer of red-staining recent thrombus.
x175 Mallory trichrome.

7.19 Endomyocardial fibrosis. Transverse short-axis section through the ventricles at papillary muscle level in chronic non-tropical endomyocardial fibrosis. A dense layer of fibrous tissue in both ventricles surrounds the papillary muscles. The apex of the right ventricle is obliterated.

7.20 Endomyocardial fibrosis. Transverse section in case shown in **7.19** taken at apical level. Dense white fibrous tissue obliterates the apex of both ventricles.

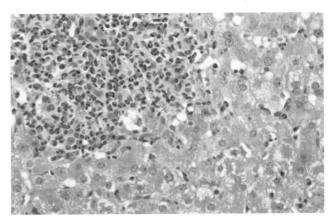

7.15 Endomyocardial fibrosis

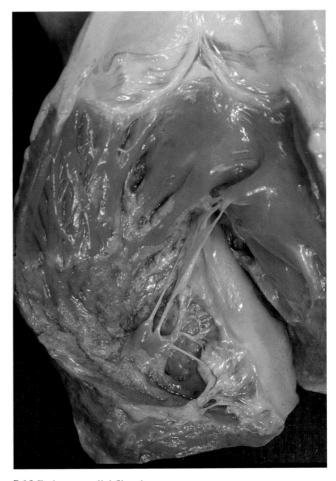

7.16 Endomyocardial fibrosis

References:

Lancet editorial. Loffler's Eosinophilic Endocarditis. Lancet 1981; 11: 1028-1028.

Olsen E G J and Spry C J F. The pathologenesis of Lofflers endomyocardial disease and its relationship to endomyocardial fibrosis. In Yu P and Goodwin J F eds. Progress in Cardiology. Philadelphia: Lea and Febiger 1979, Volume 8.

Roberts W C, Liegler D G and Carbone P P. Endomyocardial Disease and eosinophilia. A clinical and pathological spectrum. Am J Med 1969; 46: 28-42.

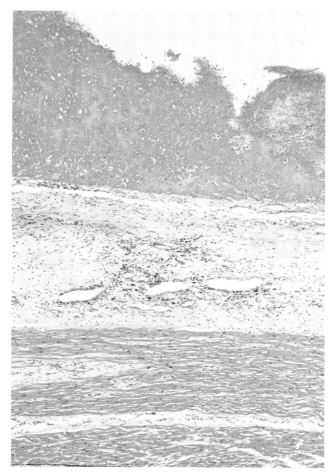

7.17 Endomyocardial fibrosis

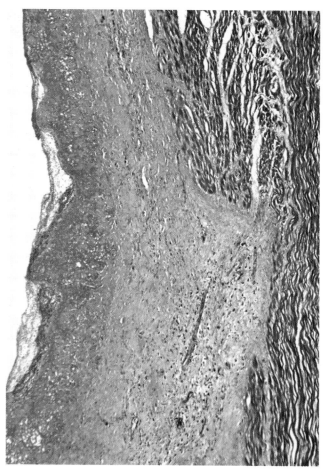

7.18 Endomyocardial fibrosis

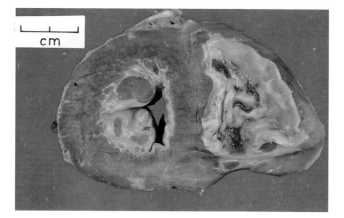

7.19 Endomyocardial fibrosis

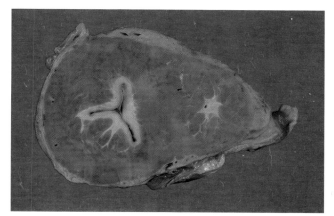

7.20 Endomyocardial fibrosis

MYOCARDITIS
(7.21 – 7.31)

The term is used by pathologists to indicate the presence of inflammatory cells in the myocardium. It is associated clinically with ventricular electrical irritability, manifested by ectopic beats, atrial fibrillation, ventricular tachycardia, and by conduction defects such as bundle-branch block or progressive atrioventricular block. These features may occur with or without evidence of failing systolic contraction in the left ventricle. The salient rhythm and conduction abnormalities have great clinical importance, in that sudden death may occur before frank cardiac failure. In mild non-fatal cases, diagnosis is very dependent on the electrocardiogram.

At a morphological level, the major criterion for diagnosis is the presence of inflammatory cells in the interstitial tissues. It is, however, the damage to myocardial cells which is responsible for the clinical manifestations. This damage may be of any degree up to total necrosis. The inflammatory infiltrate is at least in part a response to the myocardial necrosis. The difficulty in terminological separation between a cardiomyopathy and a myocarditis is directly comparable with the distinction between skeletal myopathy and myositis.

Myocarditis is due either to toxic or metabolic damage to myocardial cells or to their actual infection by organisms such as viruses or protozoa.

Now that diphtheria has vanished, it is usually assumed that most myocarditis seen today is viral in origin, although proof is seldom forthcoming. The Coxsackie virus has the best-known affinity for the myocardium, particularly in the neonatal period, both in man and experimental animals. The course of the disease in the mouse closely resembles that in man and has been extensively studied. Infection via the oral route is followed by a viremic phase shortly after which the organism can be recovered from several tissues, including heart, pancreas and brain. Myocardial necrosis develops, to be followed subsequently by a florid interstitial mononuclear cell infiltration. By this stage the virus cannot be recovered from the myocardium. In mice, there is considerable variation in cardio-selectivity and susceptibility between different strains of Coxsackie virus, but younger and newborn animals are most vulnerable in all instances. In the dog, Papova virus infection of newborn litters is now a world-wide problem and while the virus does not affect man it is of importance as a model, for within a single litter can be found a complete spectrum of puppies dying suddenly, dying in cardiac failure within a short period, or dying after a latent period of months with cardiac failure. The model may thus provide indirect evidence of the link between cardiomyopathy and viral myocarditis in man.

In man the virus most reported as a cause of myocarditis is the Coxsackie group, both in sporadic fatal cases and as a cause of death in known epidemics in the community. In myocarditis in the neonate, the proportion due to Coxsackie infection is very high. In the population as a whole, individual case reports have linked fatal myocarditis to many viruses including polio, mumps, and ECHO. Clinical surveys using ECG criteria indicate that a degree of sub-clinical myocarditis is common in all the childhood infectious fevers.

Protozoal infections in which the intracellular growth of the organisms leads to myocardial fibre death include *Trypanosoma cruzi* and *Toxoplasmosis gondii*. The former is endemic and common in parts of S. America and is again of interest in that there is an acute myocarditic phase which may be fatal but in patients who survive, a long-term progressive 'cardiomyopathy' develops due to immunological auto-immune myocardial destruction. Toxoplasma myocarditis is rare, usually ocurring in congenital infections in the neonatal period, but it has emerged as an important cause of fatality in immune-suppressed individuals, particularly recipients of cardiac transplants.

The classic cause of a toxic myocarditis is diphtheria. Here the exotoxin produced by the organism is directly cardiotoxic, producing a hyaline necrosis of myocardial fibres. Conduction fibres are particularly sensitive and this, in association with the effect of the toxin on nerve fibres, is responsible for the high incidence of heart block in acute diphtheria.

Focal myocardial necrosis with preservation of the interstitial tissues is a feature of a range of metabolic abnormalities which include hypo- and hyper-kalemia, magnesium deficiency and excess catecholamines either iatrogenic or endogenous, arising from adrenal medullary tumours. The degree of interstitial inflammatory infiltrate is rarely marked and the process is better termed a focal necrosis than a focal myocarditis.

HISTOLOGICALLY-SPECIFIC MYOCARDITIS
(7.32 – 7.46)

The alternative tissue response of the myocardium other than a mononuclear inflammatory response is the production of giant cells. An acute fulminating form of acute myocarditis usually leading to rapid death is associated with areas of necrosis in the myocardium, at the margins of which elongated multinucleated cells. An association with other auto-immune diseases, thymic tumours and sarcoidosis is recorded but most cases are only diagnosed at autopsy, and no clear pathogenesis has been established. The entity is best known as idiopathic giant-cell myocarditis.

Sarcoidosis involves the heart in a number of ways. Most common is the discovery of isolated granulomata within the myocardium when multiple routine histological blocks are taken in a case of generalized sarcoidosis in which there no cardiac symptoms. The more histological blocks of myocardium that are taken the greater will be the incidence of cardiac sarcoid. Clinically significant cardiac sarcoid occurs in two forms. In diffuse involvement, widespread myocardial fibrosis occurs, amongst which are scattered giant cell granulomata. This form is associated hemodynamically with a stiff left ventricle and a restrictive type of cardiomyopathy on clinical investigation. The other form produces a large mass of granulomatous tissue simulating an intramyocardial tumour. If such masses interrupt the conduction system sudden death may occur. In the healing phase of these masses, fibrosis develops and may lead to the formation of ventricular aneurysms.

Syphilis affects the heart by production of an inflammatory aortitis and by the formation of intramyocardial gummata. The classic site for such lesions is the upper interventricular septum, destroying the conduction system. Tuberculous involvement of the heart is rare; only isolated cases of intramyocardial tuberculomata are recorded.

The most histologically specific form of myocarditis occurs in acute rheumatic fever. The disease probably results from an immunological attack on the heart, because it shares a capsular antigen with hemolytic streptococci which have infected the body elsewhere, usually the throat. Bacteria or their antigens are not actually present in the heart.

Rheumatic fever produces a pancarditis: an acute valvulitis, myocarditis, and pericarditis. The pericarditis has the least serious sequelae; in the acute phase an effusion may be present and a pericardial rub heard. The histological appearances are non-specific and long-term effects are virtually non-existent.

The myocarditis is important because it is the cause of death in the acute phase. The myocarditis is also of interest in that it has a highly specific histological appearance characterized by formation of small giant cell granulomas known as Aschoff bodies. Aschoff bodies are very long-persisting granulomata and may be found many years after the acute attack in sites such as the left atrial appendage. With time the central zone of altered collagen vanishes and the whole complex becomes a small scar.

The importance of the valvulitis in the acute phase lies in its ability to invoke the long-term, slowly evolving valve damage that we call chronic rheumatic disease. The exact mechanism of the continuing valve damage is uncertain. It has been regarded as recurrent subclinical attacks of streptococcal infection or as a purely passive secondary change in a damaged valve. Both processes may be important in different patients. In support of the former view, the incidence of long-term damage rises with the number of attacks of acute rheumatic fever.

SPECIFIC HEART MUSCLE DISEASE (7.47 – 7.60)

This term is favoured by the WHO to indicate a 'cardiomyopathy' known to be associated with or caused by a systemic disease. The alternative approach is to regard these conditions as secondary cardiomyopathies; the use of such a term as amyloid cardiomyopathy is equally valid and widely used in the literature.

Deposition of amyloid in the heart occurs in several forms, which are to some extent distinguishable on clinical grounds. It has been realized for many years that with increasing age small deposits of material staining as amyloid appear beneath the endocardium of the left atrium. In people over 80 years of age, such deposits are the rule rather than the exception and are known as senile cardiac amyloid. They are seldom of clinical significance but may be a contributory factor to atrial fibrillation and heart failure.

In systemic amyloidosis, more significant cardiac involvement may occur; the functional effect is usually that of a restrictive cardiomyopathy due to massive involvement of the ventricles. Macroscopically the heart may be large and firm, or merely stiff and rigid to the feel without enlargement. Left atrial deposits are identical with those seen in the senile type, and atrial involvement is always heavy, leading to all foms of atrial arrhythmias. Isolated cardiac amyloidosis, identical in distribution and clinical effect to the cardiac involvement in systemic amyloid, also occurs. Recent work suggests the chemical composition of such deposits to be different from the senile form of cardiac amyloid. The earliest deposition in all forms is on the basement membrane of the myocardial cells.

In both hemochromatosis and hemosiderosis, iron is deposited in the myocardium, leading to a dilated form of cardiomyopathy. Whether endogenous or exogenous, the iron is initially deposited within myocardial fibres, subsequently being released into the interstitial tissues when myocardial muscle cell death occurs.

Alcohol has a direct toxic effect on the function of myocardial cells, and long-term alcohol abuse leads to irreversible morphological changes. In general, the hearts of alcoholic subjects at post-mortem are unduly large and have excess intramyocardial fibrosis. A small proportion of patients develop congestive cardiac failure which is clinically and pathologically indistinguishable from idiopathic dilated cardiomyopathy.

All forms of skeletal muscular dystrophy and many of the hereditary neuromyopathy syndromes have an appreciable incidence of concomitant heart muscle disease. This may even predate or predominate over obvious skeletal involvement. In the majority of cases a congestive type of cardiomyopathy occurs without specific morphological distinguishing features within the heart. Taken overall, conduction defects are rather more comon than with idiopathic cardiomyopathy. The incidence of cardiac involvement is highest in myotonic dystrophy. In Friedreich's ataxia, the cardiac involvement has more affinity with hypertrophic cardiomyopathy.

In children, glycogen storage disease produces a characteristic histological picture in the myocardium. Macroscopically the heart is hypertrophied often with asymmetrical septal hypertrophy simulating hypertrophic cardiomyopathy. A rare form of infantile cardiomyopathy occurs where lipid is present within myocardial cells.

In all types of mucopolysaccharidosis, histiocytic cells containing the abnormal mucin are present predominantly in the connective tissue of the valve rings, valve cusps and the intimal of small coronary arteries.

MYOCARDIAL DEGENERATION
(7.61 – 7.67)

Fatty infiltration of the myocardium (that is, adipose tissue between myocardial fibres) is extremely common in the right ventricle, increasing in frequency with age. Fatty degeneration is rarer but equally non-specific and analogous to fatty change in the liver.

Metastatic myocardial calcification occurs in a wide range of conditions associated with hypercalcemia in renal failure. Calcium is deposited in individual cells, immediately adjacent cells being normal. Basophilic mucoid degeneration is the accumulation of amorphous blue material within isolated myocardial cells. It has no specificity, being found to some degree in many hearts from old people. It does occur in myxedema but again is not specific. The change is also present to some extent in many cardiomyopathies.

ENDOCARDIAL FIBROELASTOSIS
(7.68 – 7.71)

This entity is usually considered amongst the cardiomyopathies, although its position is an anomalous one. The characteristic feature is endocardial thickening in the left atrium and ventricle with a smooth porcelain-like surface. The histological pattern is of endocardial thickening containing multiple parallel elastic laminae. The process is more likely to be a response of the young endocardium rather than a specific disease process.

The endocardial fibroelastosis associated with left-sided congenital defects, including aortic stenosis, ventricular septal defects and coarctation is usually distinguished from primary fibroelastosis not associated with any other anomaly. Fibroelastosis is also associated with hypoplasia of the left side of the heart which gives a tiny chamber lined by thick white endocardium. This is the so-called contracted type of endocardial fibroelastosis. Primary fibroelastosis may or may not be associated with myocardial scarring. In some instances the distinction between a dilated type of congestive cardiomyopathy and endocardial fibroelastosis in a young child is arbitrary.

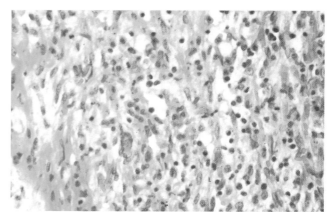

7.21 Viral myocarditis

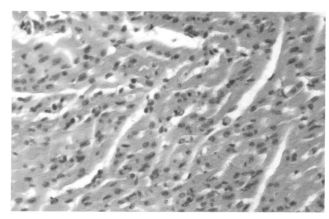

7.22 Viral myocarditis

7.21, 7.22 Acute viral myocarditis. (7.21) Fatal viral myocarditis due to Coxsackie infection in a neonate. Virus was recovered from both mother and infant. In the myocardium of the infant the loss of myocardial muscle cells is best appreciated by comparison with a section of normal age-matched myocardium **(7.22)**. In the section from the infant with myocarditis **(7.21)** there is preservation of the interstitial tissues, with an increase of macrophages and some mononuclear cells.
x275 Hematoxylin and eosin.

References:

Billingham M E. Some recent advances in cardiac pathology. Human Pathology 1979; 10: 367-387.

Silver M M and Silver M D. The Cardiomyopathies. In Silver M D ed. Cardiovascular Pathology. New York: Churchill Livingstone 1983; 489-516.

Woodruff J F. Viral myocarditis – a review. Am J Pathol 1980; 101: 425-484.

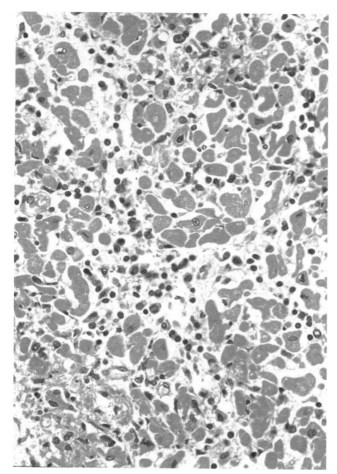

7.23 Viral myocarditis

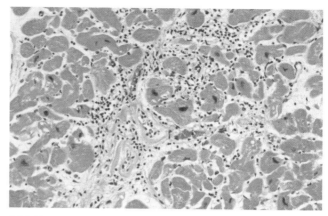

7.24 Chronic myocarditis

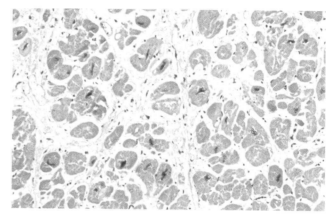

7.25 Chronic myocarditis

7.23   Acute viral myocarditis. Viral myocarditis due to Coxsackie infection. In this case muscle fibre loss is less striking but there is a heavy interstitial infiltrate of lymphocytes, plasma cells and some eosinophils. Many of the muscle fibres are swollen, others are hypereosinophilic. x425 Hematoxylin and eosin.

7.24, 7.25   Chronic myocarditis or dilated cardiomyopathy. (7.24) Myocarditis of unknown etiology in a patient dying a year after the sudden onset with fever of cardiac failure. There is irregular hypertrophy of myocardial fibres and an interstitial infiltrate of chronic inflammatory cells. An adjacent histological section **(7.25)** showed appearances which would be interpreted as dilated cardiomyopathy in that inflammatory cells are absent. It is this type of clinical and pathological case which illustrates the vague borderline between idiopathic congestive cardiomyopathy and myocarditis.
x350 Hematoxylin and eosin.

7.26 Myocarditis due to toxoplasmosis. Fatal congenital toxoplasmosis in an infant. Intracellular organisms are seen within one muscle fibre. Characteristically there is no inflammatory response in this area. The inflammatory response is assumed to occur after the infected cells die or as in Chagas disease to be an auto-immune response not directly aimed at the organisms. Similar appearances are found in immune-suppressed individuals who develop toxoplasmosis of the myocardium.
x325 Hematoxylin and eosin.

7.27 Diphtheritic myocarditis. Fatal diphtheritic myocarditis in which toxin produced by the organism induces myocardial necrosis. There is myocardial necrosis with interstitial proliferation of fibroblasts and an infiltrate of mononuclear cells. The feature which suggests, but is by no means specific for, a toxin-mediated lesion is the hyaline necrosis of individual myocardial cells (arrows).
x225 Hematoxylin and eosin.

7.28 Catecholamine-induced myocardial damage. Focal area of myocardial fibre loss in a patient dying with a functional adrenal medullary tumour. There are empty sarcolemmal sheaths in the form of round spaces within which have appeared macrophages. The lesion progresses to collapse of the interstitial tissue, leaving a tiny focal scar often containing some residual lipofuscin. Massive elevation of catecholamine levels may lead to larger confluent areas of necrosis and intramyocardial hemorrhage. While often called 'focal myocarditis' the lesions resulting from increased catecholamine levels and many other metabolic processes are in reality focal areas of necrosis.
x225 Hematoxylin and eosin.

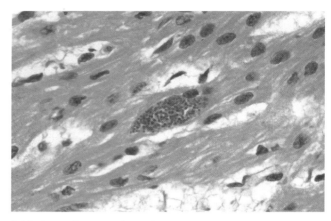

7.26 Myocarditis: toxoplasmosis

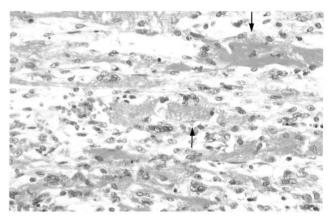

7.27 Diphtheritic myocarditis

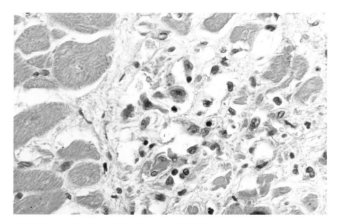

7.28 Catecholamine-induced myocardial damage

7.29 Acute giant-cell myocarditis. Idiopathic giant-cell myocarditis in a young woman dying within a few hours of developing fever, tachycardia and palpitations. The myocardium shows irregular serpiginous areas of pale necrosis. The etiology of this very fulminating form of myocarditis is unknown.

7.30 Acute giant-cell myocarditis. Histological section through the margin of an area of myocardial necrosis in idiopathic giant-cell myocarditis. Numerous giant cells are present in apposition to the ends of remaining myocardial cells.
x225 Hematoxylin and eosin.

7.31 Acute giant-cell myocarditis. Higher-power view of the giant cells in idiopathic giant-cell myocarditis. The giant cells are multinucleated, with nuclei resembling myocardial fibre nuclei rather than those of macrophages. In addition the cells appear to contain myofibrils and lipofuscin. These features have been used to suggest that the giant cells are myogenic in origin although there is also evidence of histiocytic origin. In addition to the giant cells there is fibroblastic proliferation and a considerable infiltrate of other chronic inflammatory cells, prominent amongst which are eosinophils.
x275 Hematoxylin and eosin.

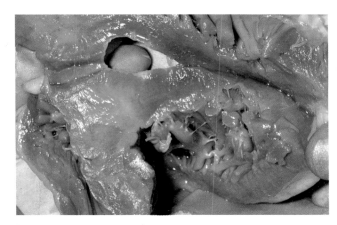

7.29 Giant-cell myocarditis

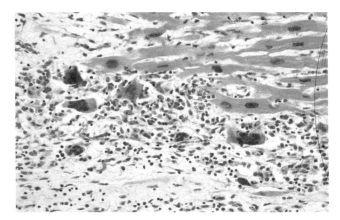

7.30 Giant-cell myocarditis

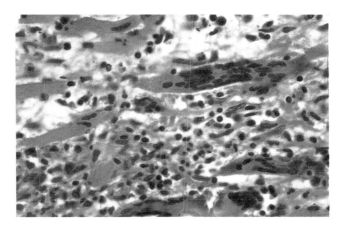

7.31 Giant-cell myocarditis

Reference:

Becker A E. Myocarditis. In Silver M D ed. Cardiovascular Pathology. New York: Churchill Livingstone 1983; 469-489.

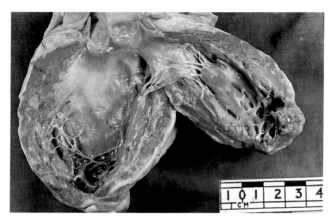

7.32 Myocardial sarcoidosis

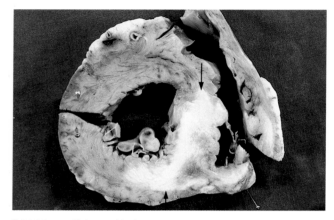

7.34 Myocardial sarcoidosis

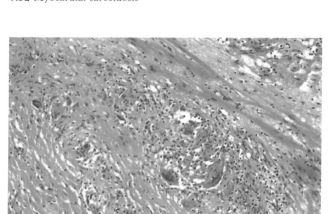

7.33 Myocardial sarcoidosis

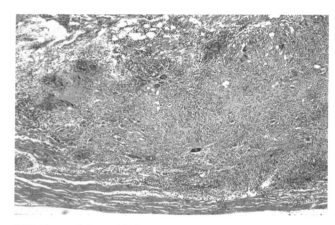

7.35 Myocardial sarcoidosis

7.32 Myocardial sarcoidosis: diffuse form. Cardiac involvement in a patient with pulmonary sarcoid who developed a restrictive type of cardiomyopathy. The myocardium of the left ventricle is diffusely scarred throughout but the heart is not markedly enlarged nor the ventricle dilated.

7.33 Myocardial sarcoidosis. Histological section through an area of myocardial fibrosis showing well-formed, but loosely arranged, follicular giant-cell granulomata.
x250 Hematoxylin and eosin.

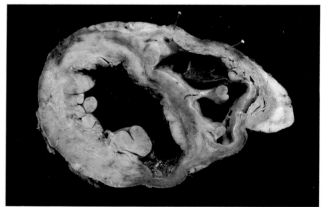

7.36 Myocardial sarcoidosis

References:

Roberts W C, McAllister H A and Ferrans V J. Sarcoidosis of the heart – a clinicopathological review of 35 necropsy patients and review of 78 previously described cases. Am J Med 1977; 63: 86-108.

Silverman K T, Hutchins G M and Bulkley B H. Cardiac Sarcoid: A clinicopathological study of 84 unselected patients with systemic sarcoidosis. Circulation 1978; 58: 1204-1211.

7.34 Myocardial sarcoidosis: localized form. Cross-section of the left and right ventricles in a patient with pulmonary sarcoid who developed heart block. A discrete solid white fibrous mass (arrows) replaces the posterior third of the interventricular septum and spreads into the posterior wall of both the right and left ventricles.

7.35 Myocardial sarcoidosis: localized form. Histological section through the fibrous mass showing it to be largely composed of an infiltrate of chronic inflammatory cells amid connective tissue. At the margins there are follicular giant-cell granulomata.
x125 Hematoxylin and eosin.

7.36 Myocardial sarcoidosis: localized form. Short axis transverse slice across the ventricles. There is a linear fibrous scar in the interventricular septum with a localized aneurysm of the posterior wall of the left ventricle. Giant-cell granulomas were scanty which is typical of the healed phase of localized cardiac sarcoid.

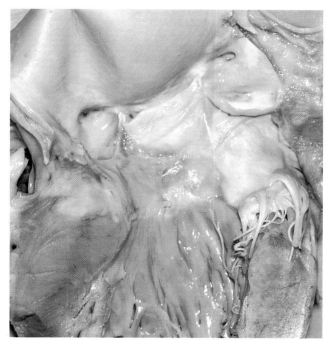
7.37 Cardiac syphilis

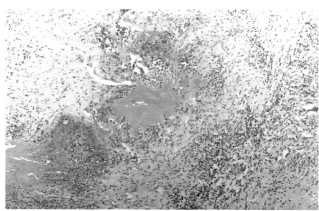
7.38 Cardiac syphilis

7.37 Cardiac syphilis. A gumma replaces the upper interventricular septum extending up to the aortic valve. From a patient with complete heart block and tertiary syphilis. This is the most common site for a cardiac gumma and it destroys the conduction system. It is quite different from syphilitic aortitis although if the gumma reaches the base of the valve cusps aortic regurgitation may develop.

7.38 Cardiac syphilis. Histology of the gumma showing a central area of structured fibrinoid necrosis at the margins of which is fibrous tissue heavily infiltrated with plasma cells.
x125 Hematoxylin and eosin.

7.39 Cardiac syphilis. Higher power view of a gumma showing the necrosis in which the tissue outlines are preserved, and the rather small non-specific giant cells of syphilis.
x95 Hematoxylin and eosin.

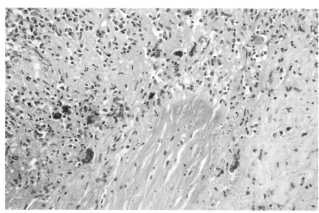
7.39 Cardiac syphilis

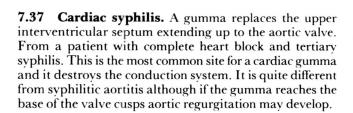

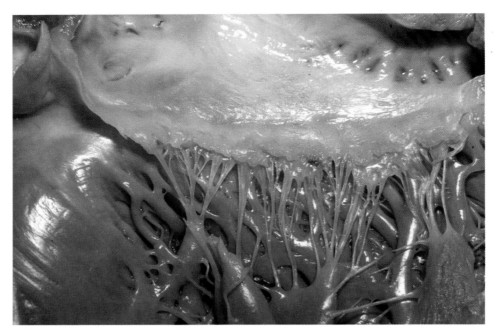

7.40 Acute rheumatic valvulitis

7.40   Acute rheumatic valvulitis. The mitral valve in an adolescent dying of acute rheumatic fever. There is a row of small sessile vegetations along the closure line on the posterior cusp. This closure line, where the cusps appose, is 2-3mm above the free edge of the cusp. The vegetations are fawn in colour, being composed almost entirely of platelets. They do not reach sizes larger than those shown here and do not lead to emboli. The distribution and size of the vegetations distinguish the condition from infective endocarditis.

7.41   Acute rheumatic valvulitis. Histological section across the valve shown in **7.40**. The valve has increased cellularity and there is surface deposition of small thrombi (arrow).
x25 Hematoxylin and eosin.

7.42   Acute rheumatic myocarditis: Aschoff body. Histological section showing an active Aschoff body in the interstitial tissue. It is an oval mass of connective tissue containing small giant cells and other mononuclear cells. The position in a small fibrous septa in the myocardium is typical.
x150 Hematoxylin and eosin.

7.43   Acute rheumatic myocarditis: Aschoff body. Histological section showing a higher-power view of the cells in the Aschoff body. There is a central area of amorphous collagen surrounding which is a mixture of giant cells with vesicular nuclei and prominent nucleoli. These are Aschoff giant cells. Other cells have open nuclei with a

very pronounced central chromatin bar (Anitschkow cells) (arrow). The origin of these cells has always been controversial, with evidence both for a myocardial and for a connective tissue origin being published.
x375 Hematoxylin and eosin.

7.44   Acute rheumatic myocarditis. Sub-endocardial tissue containing numerous Aschoff bodies forming a continuous line of still-discrete entities. This subendocardial location, particularly in the left atrium, is typical.
x95 Hematoxylin and eosin.

7.45   Acute rheumatic myocarditis. Sub-endocardial tissue in a fatal florid case of acute rheumatic fever. There is a linear area of intensely eosinophilic collagen around which are histiocytic cells arranged in regular rows. This structure is a form of giant Aschoff body but rather reminiscent of a rheumatoid nodule. It is only seen in extremely florid cases from areas of the world where acute rheumatic disease is still rampant.
x80 Hematoxylin and eosin.

7.46   Healing rheumatic myocarditis. Healing Aschoff body with interstitial fibrosis embedded in which are a few small giant cells with dark pyknotic nuclei. Aschoff bodies may remain in this state for many years. They cannot, therefore, be used to indicate rheumatic activity, merely that the patient has had acute rheumatic fever at some time in the past. After many years the Aschoff body becomes replaced by an acellular fibrous scar.
x150 Hematoxylin and eosin.

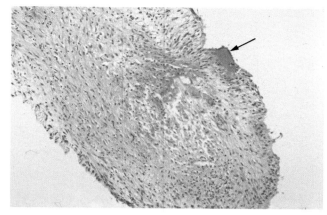

7.41 Acute rheumatic valvulitis

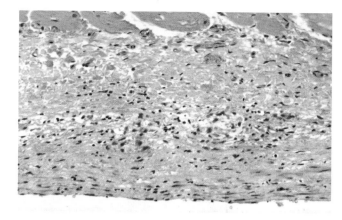

7.44 Acute rheumatic myocarditis

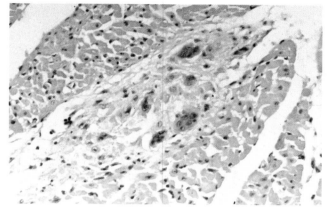

7.42 Aschoff body

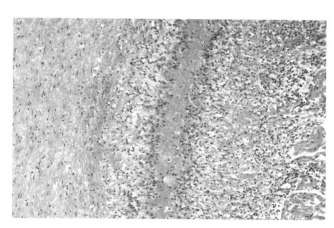

7.45 Acute rheumatic myocarditis

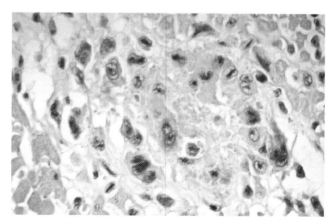

7.43 Aschoff body

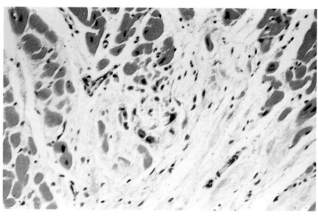

7.46 Healing rheumatic myocarditis

7.47 Amyloid disease of the heart. A formalin-fixed specimen of the heart to show brown nodules of amyloid beneath the endocardium of the left atrium. The nodules, typical of senile cardiac amyloid, are more easily recognized in fixed than in fresh tissue.

7.48 Amyloid disease of the heart. Amyloid deposits appearing as nodules of amorphous pink material in the small arteries of a patient with senile cardiac amyloid who was clinically asymptomatic.
x225 Hematoxylin and eosin.

7.49 Amyloid disease of the heart. Amyloid deposits staining paler than the uninvolved myocardium in the left ventricle of a patient dying of primary cardiac amyloid. The pale-staining amyloid material forms a lattice or honeycomb within which are embedded remnants of myocardial fibres. The pattern of deposition makes amyloid instantly distinguishable from collagen even without the use of specific stains.
x275 Hematoxylin and eosin.

7.50 Amyloid deposition in the myocardium: ultrastructure. Electronmicrogram of a left ventricular biopsy from a patient with restrictive cardiomyopathy. A layer of fibrillary amyloid material (arrows) is evenly spread along the external surface of a myocardial muscle cell.

7.51 Amyloid disease of the heart. Advanced cardiac amyloid with complete loss of myocardial fibres and formation of large amorphous masses of amyloid material which are invoking a giant-cell response.
x150 Hematoxylin and eosin.

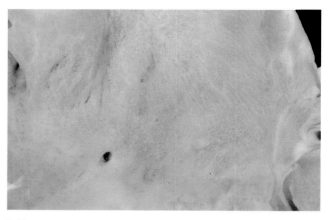

7.47 Amyloid disease

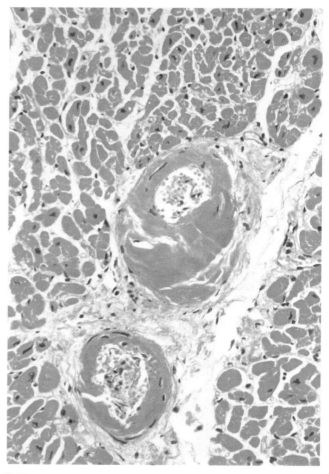

7.48 Amyloid disease

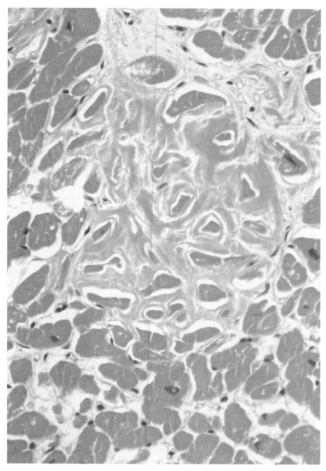

7.49 Amyloid disease

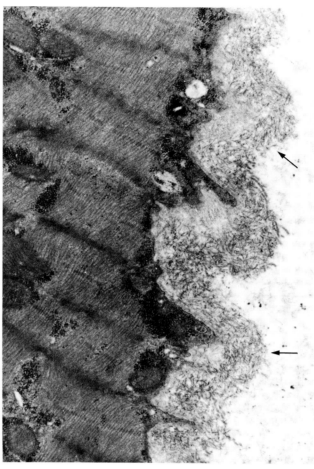

7.50 Amyloid: ultrastructure

References:

Cutler D J, Isner J M, Bracey A W, Hufnagel C A, Conrad P W, Roberts W C, Kerwin D M and Weintraub A M. Hemochromatosis heart disease: an unemphasized cause of potentially reversible restrictive cardiomyopathy. Am J Med 1980; 69: 923-928.

Dabestani A, Child J S, Henze E, Perloff J K, Schon H, Figueroa W G, Schelbert H R and Thessomboon S. Primary hemochromatosis: Anatomic and physiologic characteristics of the cardiac ventricles and their response to phlebotomy. Am J Cardiol 1984; 54: 153-160.

Roberts W C and Waller B F. Cardiac amyloidosis causing cardiac dysfunction analysis of 54 necropsy patients. Am J Cardiol 1983; 52: 137-146.

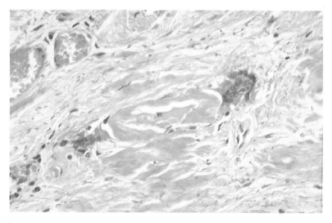

7.51 Amyloid disease

7.52   The myocardium in iron storage disorders.
The myocardium from a patient with hemochromatosis.
Brown pigment is distributed throughout the cytoplasm
of the myocardial cells although there is a greater con-
centration of granules in the perinuclear zone. There is
fine fibrosis but no iron pigment is present in the interstitial space.
x300 Hematoxylin and eosin.

7.53   The myocardium in iron overload. The myocardium from the same patient as in **7.52** stained to
demonstrate iron as blue granules in all the myocardial
cells. The amount of iron present is greater than would be
anticipated from the ordinary hematoxylin and eosin-
stained sections.
x300 Perls' stain.

7.54   The myocardium in iron overload. The myocardium from a patient in the late stage of iron deposition.
There is dense interstitial fibrosis containing large granular deposits of iron which have been released by death of
myocardial cells.
x300 Hematoxylin and eosin.

**7.55   Cardiac involvement in familial skeletal myo-
pathy.** The heart is from a patient with a familial skeletal
myopathy who had an abnormal electrocardiogram and
died suddenly at the age of 22. The specimen is a transverse slice across both ventricles which has been stained to
demonstrate succinic dehydrogenase activity (red). No
recent necrosis is present but there is a band of subpericardial fibrous scarring (white) on the posterior wall of the
left ventricle. The coronary arteries were entirely normal.
The postero-basal portion of the ventricle is the favoured
site for scarring in some forms of skeletal myopathy. The
reasons are unknown.

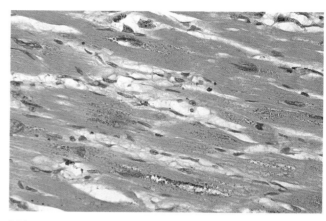

7.52 Iron storage disease

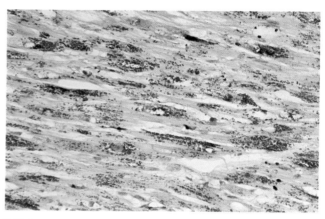

7.53 Iron overload

7.56   Cardiac involvement in skeletal myopathy. The
myocardium from a patient with a familial skeletal myopathy. Broad bands of fibrosis separate groups of myocardial fibres. The coronary arteries were normal. The
cause of the myocardial fibrosis is obscure; some
authorities have implicated abnormalities of the muscle of
the medial coats of the small intra-myocardial coronary
arteries ('small vessel disease') but these are somewhat
inconstant and not always present even when scarring is
present.
x45 Picro-Mallory.

7.57   Glycogen storage disease. Glycogen storage
disease in an infant dying before one year of age. There are
areas in which the myocardial fibres are empty and vacuolated; in contrast adjacent myocardial fibres are more
normal. The patchy distribution is common in the disease.
x125 Hematoxylin and eosin.

7.58   Glycogen storage disease. Higher-power view of
the abnormal myocardial fibres in glycogen storage
disease shown in **7.57**. The myocardial fibres appear
empty, the glycogen having been dissolved out in fixation
and processing of the tissue. The cells contain very scanty
peripheral myofibrils.
x350 Hematoxylin and eosin.

Reference:

Perloff J K. Cardiomyopathy associated with heredofamilial
    neuromyopathic disease. Modern Concepts of Cardiovascular
    Disease 1971; 40: 23-26.

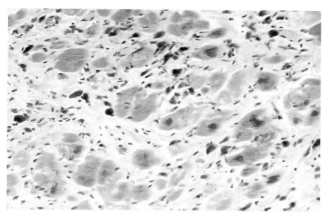

7.54 Iron overload

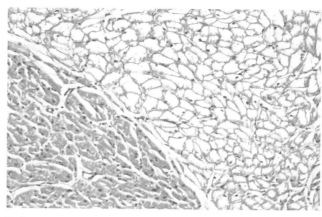

7.57 Glycogen storage disease

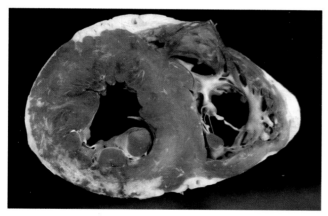

7.55 Familial skeletal myopathy

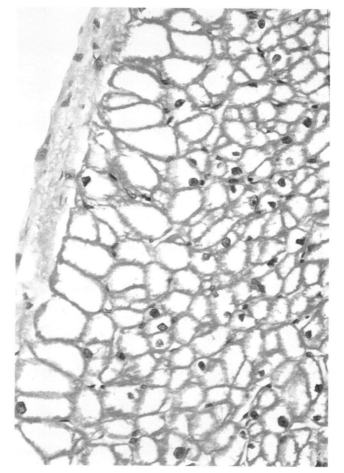

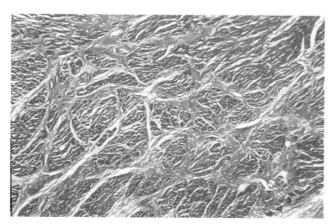

7.56 Skeletal myopathy

7.58 Glycogen storage disease

7.59 Cardiac mucopolysaccharidosis. The mitral valve from a child dying with Hurler's syndrome. At this low magnification the connective tissue of the valve fibrosa appears honeycombed rather than solid.
x14 Hematoxylin and eosin.

7.60 Cardiac mucopolysaccharidosis. At higher-power the honeycombing of the valve fibrosa shown in **7.59** can be seen to be due to infiltration by histiocytic cells with clear cytoplasm.
x75 Hematoxlin and eosin.

7.61 Fatty degeneration of the myocardium. Fatty degeneration of the myocardium of a diabetic patient who was also alcoholic. Every muscle cell contains numerous fine lipid droplets evenly distributed throughout the cell.
x350 Sudan Red.

7.62 Myocardial calcification. Calcification of an individual myocardial muscle cell in a patient with hyperparathyroidism. A single cell has become deeply basophilic from the presence of punctate and linear deposits of calcium. Immediately adjacent cells are normal.
x350 Hematoxylin and eosin.

7.63 Myocardial calcification. Myocardial calcification in a patient in chronic renal failure. There is a large area of calcification within which the ghost outlines of the original myocardial cells can be made out.
x75 Hematoxylin and eosin.

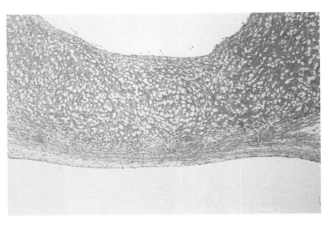

7.59 Cardiac mucopolysaccharidosis

7.64 Myocardial calcification. Massive subendocardial calcification in an infant. On one side of the section the myocardium is normal; on the other side the tissue outlines are retained but all the muscle fibres are calcified and there is a giant-cell response to the calcific material. While this picture can occur in infants with enhanced calcification due to renal failure, many cases have no biochemical abnormality and are thought to result from viral myocarditis. A similar change also occurs with anomalous coronary arteries. It thus appears that infants have a greater capacity to calcify areas of myocardial necrosis.
x60 Hematoxylin and eosin.

7.65 Mucoid degeneration of myocardial cells. In one of the myocardial muscle fibres is an oval perinuclear vacuole which contains slightly basophilic mucoid material. The change is totally nonspecific, occurring with increasing age in normal hearts.
x450 Hematoxylin and eosin.

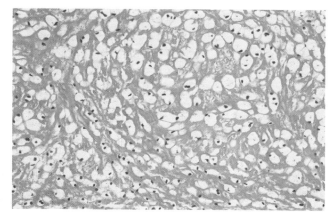

7.60 Cardiac mucopolysaccharidosis

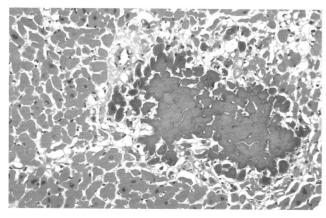

7.63 Myocardial calcification

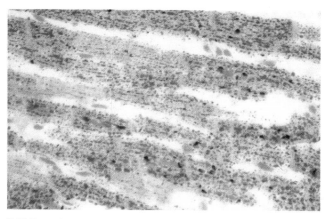

7.61 Fatty degeneration

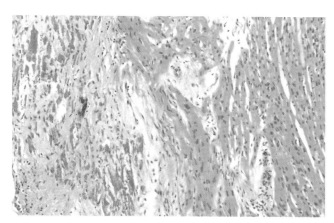

7.64 Myocardial calcification

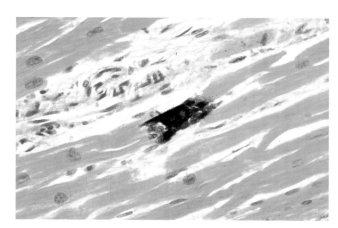

7.62 Myocardial calcification

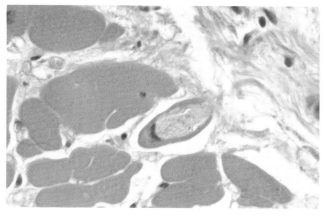

7.65 Mucoid degeneration

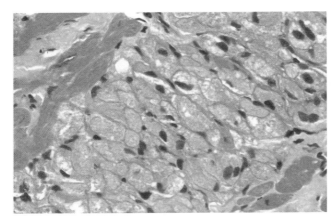

7.66 Isolated cardiac lipoidosis

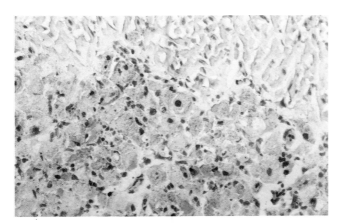

7.67 Isolated cardiac lipoidosis

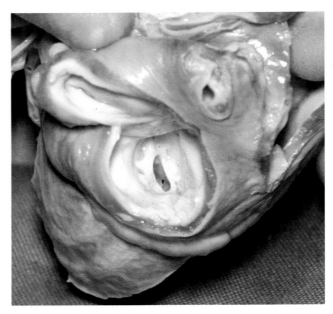

7.68 Endocardial fibroelastosis

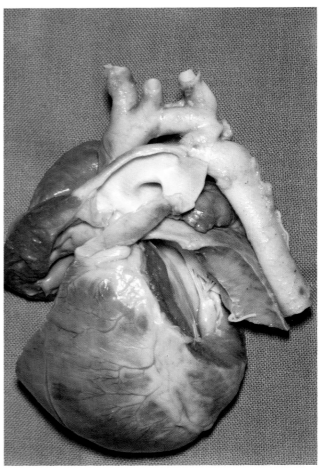

7.69 Hypoplastic left heart syndrome

7.66 Isolated cardiac lipoidosis or 'histiocytoid' cardiomyopathy. The infant died of intractable ventricular tachycardia. There is a small focus of eosinophilic and relatively normal myocardial cells but most muscle cells have been converted into paler-staining cells with slightly granular cytoplasm resembling histiocytes. The pathogenesis of this change is unknown.
x275 Hematoxylin and eosin.

7.67 Isolated cardiac lipoidosis or 'histiocytoid' cardiomyopathy. Focus of histiocytic myocardial cells stained to demonstrate their lipid content as orange-red droplets. Adjacent myocardial cells are free of lipid. There is considerable disagreement over the origin of the lipid-containing cells. They have been regarded as true histiocytes or as transformed myocardial muscle cells and it has also been proposed that they are of conduction fibre (Purkinje cell) origin.
x225 Sudan.

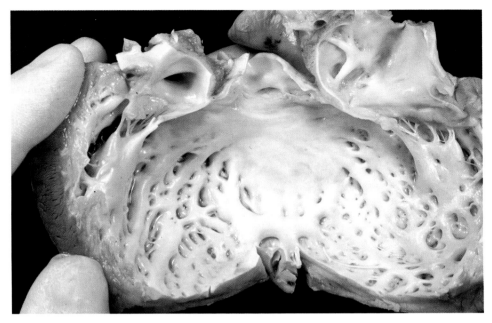

7.70 Dilated endocardial fibroelastosis

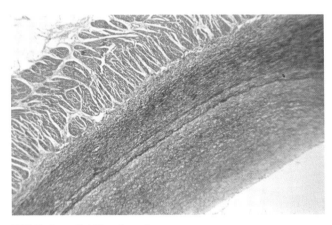

7.71 Endocardial fibroelastosis

7.68 Endocardial fibroelastosis in the left atrium. The atrial cavity is tiny with a thick white opaque endocardium which extends down into the mitral valve whose orifice is small. Ths form of fibroelastosis is part of the hypoplastic left heart syndrome. The mitral valve could also be regarded as congenitally stenotic although it is better thought of as a 'miniaturized' valve.

7.69 Hypoplastic left heart syndrome. The same specimen as **7.68.** The left ventricle is tiny, with a thick white endocardium. This can be regarded as the contracted type of fibroelastosis. The right ventricle is vast as a result of pulmonary hypertension which develops in these cases. The tiny left atrium acts physiologically as mitral stenosis leading to high pulmonary venous pressures and subsequent arterial hypertension.

7.70 Dilated form of endocardial fibroelastosis. The left ventricle is dilated, with a thick white porcelain-like endocardium. The subendocardial myocardium is scarred. This heart could be regarded as a dilated endocardial fibroelastosis or as a dilated cardiomyopathy in a child.

7.71 Endocardial fibroelastosis in left atrium. The endocardium is thicker than the myocardial layer and contains numerous parallel elastic laminae.
x40 Elastic-van Gieson.

References:

Bruton D, Herdson P B and Beecroft D M O. Histiocytoid cardiomyopathy of infancy: an unexplained myofibre degeneration. Pathology 1977; 9: 123-125.

McGregor C G A, Gibson A and Caves P. Infantile cardiomyopathy with histiocytoid change in cardiac muscle cells: successful surgical intervention and prolonged survival. Am J Cardiol 1984; 53: 982-982.

Neill C A and Ursell P. Endocardial Fibroelastosis and left heart hypoplasia revisited. International Journal of Cardiology 1984; 5: 547-549.

Silver M M, Burns J E, Sethi R K and Rowe R D. Oncocytic cardiomyopathy in an infant with oncocytosis in exocrine and endocrine glands. Human Pathology 1980; 11: 598-605.

CHAPTER 8

Cor Pulmonale

A strict definition of this term is of prime importance. Cor pulmonale is defined as right ventricular hypertrophy consequent upon pulmonary hypertension which is caused by diseases of the structure and function of the lung and its blood vessels. It is mandatory to exclude cases where the lung disease is the result of processes primarily affecting the left side of the heart or of congenital heart disease. Thus the pulmonary hypertension of mitral valve stenosis or of a left-to-right shunt in an atrial septal defect is *not* designated as cor pulmonale. Some semantic difficulties still arise; on occasion the left-sided heart disease is not apparent in life, and an erroneous clinical diagnosis of cor pulmonale is made. Another misconception arises over clinical usage of the term acute cor pulmonale for patients with large pulmonary emboli and whose subsequent clinical and pathological features have nothing in common with chronic cor pulmonale.

Pulmonary hypertension in cor pulmonale arises from three basic processes which may occur in isolation or combine in any individual patient. The first of these is purely functional: an alteration in the calibre of pulmonary arterioles due to medial muscle contraction. The second is the development of intimal proliferation in the arterioles leading to vascular obstruction, which changes a case of reversible pulmonary hypertension to one which is irreversible. Finally, there may be widespread destruction of the pulmonary capillary bed.

The best example of purely functional pulmonary hypertension is seen in subjects living at high altitude and is reversible when they return to lower levels. Patients with restricted chest movement due to extreme obesity or neuromuscular disease also develop hypoxia and thus pulmonary hypertension. In patients with pure chronic bronchitis, the cause of pulmonary hypertension is hypoxia resulting from airway obstruction and lack of respiratory drive. Diseases such as emphysema and pulmonary fibrosis, whether secondary to tuberculosis, sarcoidosis or an industrial disease, lead both to perfusion/ventilation mismatching within the lung and to an actual destruction of the vascular bed.

Primary vascular disease of the pulmonary vessels themselves arises in three instances, all of which are rare. Firstly, primary arterial pulmonary hypertension results from what is assumed to be initially spasm followed by irreversible intimal damage. What initiates the arterial spasm is unknown. The condition is more common in women, and some cases have been linked with use of an anti-appetite drug Aminorex or contaminated cooking oils. Secondly, thrombo-embolic pulmonary hypertension arises in patients who repeatedly throw small emboli into the lungs over a long period. Characteristically the source of these small emboli in the legs or pelvis is not clinically obvious and large pulmonary emboli are unusual. Finally there is a very rare form of pulmonary arterial hypertension which follows pulmonary venous hypertension due to a veno-occlusive disease of the lung.

The macroscopic and microscopic effects on the heart and pulmonary vessels are identical, whatever the cause of pulmonary hypertension. The right ventricle becomes hypertrophied as judged by the right ventricular muscle mass. In extreme cases the right ventricle may exceed the left in size. Lesser degrees of right ventricular hypertrophy are not easy to recognize, and ventricular wall thickness is a notoriously unreliable parameter. No other visual assessment made by pathologists at autopsy is so subjective. The only accurate method is to weigh the isolated right ventricle.

In patients with extreme pulmonary hypertension the foramen ovale may bulge into the left atrium as an 'aneurysm', and occasionally a small right-to-left shunt develops. Some thickening of the anterior cusp of the tricuspid valve and pulmonary valve cusps occurs. The main pulmonary artery dilates and shows development of plaques of atheroma. This does not usually progress to become complicated by mural thrombus.

In pulmonary hypertension the vascular changes have been described in an ascending scale of six grades by Heath and Edwards, but these are actually a continuous spectrum. The medial changes consist of both hypertrophy of medial smooth muscle and its extension peripherally into vessels that do not normally have medial muscle. Assessment of medial muscle hypertrophy thus requires both considerable experience and detailed measurement of medial thickness in relation to the size of the vessel.

The intima undergoes concentric fibrous thickening until it virtually obliterates the lumen. This advanced change can be recognized as a 'pruning' of the peripheral vascular bed in angiograms. As well as being characterized by intimal fibrosis, the final two grades of pulmonary vascular changes have more complex lesions, usually described as angiomatoid, aneurysmal or plexiform. A small minority of cases may develop fibrinoid necrosis of vessel walls.

The most severe degrees of pulmonary vascular change do not usually occur outside primary pulmonary hypertension. The exceptions are that grade five and six vascular changes develop in left-to-right shunts in congenital heart disease as part of the Eisenmenger syndrome and also in the pulmonary hypertension arising very early in life as a result of endocardial fibroelastosis of the left atrium. Neither of these conditions is, of course, cor pulmonale by definition. Thrombo-embolic pulmonary hypertension produces lesions in the pulmonary vessels which, for all practical purposes, are microscopically indistinguishable from other forms of primary pulmonary hypertension. The presence of small fibrin thrombi and revascularization patterns, while in theory being more in favour of thrombo-embolic disease, have not proved to be so in practice. This may well indicate that even in non-embolic primary pulmonary hypertension, vascular thrombosis plays a major role.

References:

Fulton R M, Hutchinson E C and Morgan Jones A. Ventricular weight in cardiac hypertrophy. Br Heart J 1952; 14: 413-420.

Heath D and Edwards J E. The pathology of hypertensive pulmonary vascular disease. A description of six grades of structural changes in the pulmonary arteries with special reference to congenital cardiac septal defects. Circulation 1958; 18: 533-547.

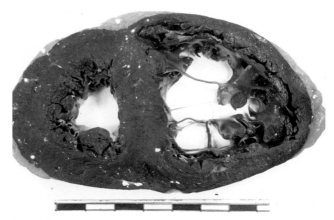

8.1 Right ventricular hypertrophy

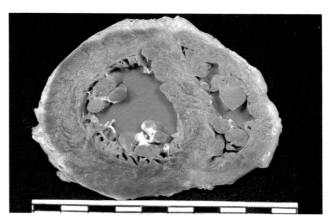

8.2 Right ventricular hypertrophy

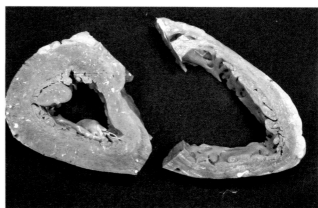

8.3 Fulton technique: ventricular hypertrophy

8.1 Right ventricular hypertrophy due to pulmonary hypertension. Gross right ventricular hypertrophy in a case of primary pulmonary hypertension. Short axis transection of ventricles. The right ventricular mass weighed 116g, the left only 109g. This degree of right ventricular hypertrophy is so gross that recognition is relatively easy.

8.2 Right ventricular hypertrophy in chronic bronchitis. A more usual degree of right ventricular hypertrophy in a case of cor pulmonale due to chronic bronchitis. The right ventricular mass was 85g, the left 160g, giving a ratio of left-to-right ventricular weights of 1.9. In this particular case, wall thickness measurement of the right ventricle is elevated.

8.3 Fulton techniques for assessment of ventricular hypertrophy. In the Fulton technique for estimation of isolated ventricular weights, the atria and all the epicardial fat are removed. The ventricles are then separated and, as these slices show, the interventricular septum is taken as being part of the left ventricle.

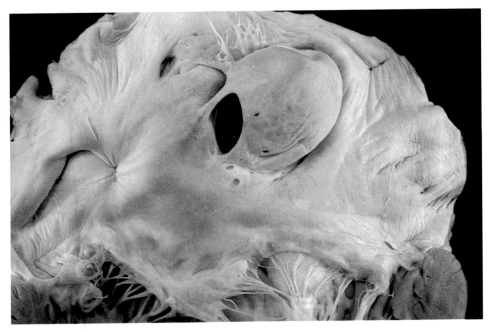

8.4 Right to left arterial shunt

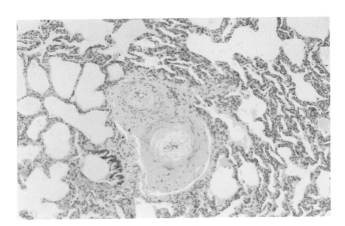

8.5 Vascular changes: pulmonary hypertension

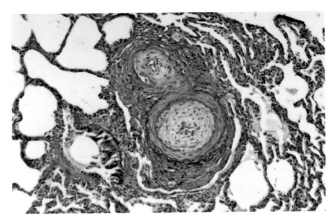

8.6 Vascular changes: pulmonary hypertension

8.4   Right to left arterial shunt in cor pulmonale.
The atrial septum viewed from the left side in a patient with cor pulmonale. The foramen ovale has bulged into the left atrium, and a small shunt had developed through a defect at the margin.

8.5, 8.6   Vascular changes in severe pulmonary hypertension. In the hematoxylin and eosin-stained section **8.5**, the arterial wall is obviously thickened and the lumen very small. When stained by the elastic-van Gieson method **(8.6)**, which demonstrates the internal elastic lamina clearly, it can be seen that most of the thickening is from intimal fibrosis.
8.5 x60 Hematoxylin and eosin.
8.6 x60 Elastic-van Gieson.

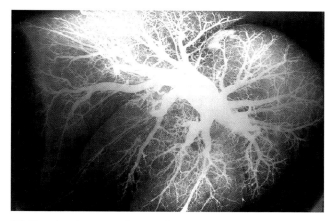

8.7 Vascular changes: pulmonary hypertension

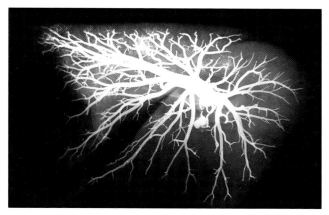

8.8 Vascular changes: pulmonary hypertension

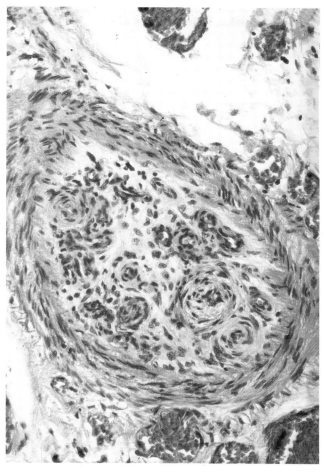

8.9 Vascular changes: primary pulmonary hypertension

8.7 Vascular changes in severe pulmonary hypertension. Post-mortem pulmonary arteriogram in a subject with a normal peripheral pulmonary arterial tree. Small vessels fill far out into the distal lung fields.

8.8 Vascular changes in severe pulmonary hypertension. Post-mortem angiogram of pulmonary artery in a patient with primary pulmonary hypertension. The small peripheral branches do not fill, having been obliterated by the intimal changes. In clinical terminology the small pulmonary arteries have been 'pruned'.

8.9 Vascular changes in primary pulmonary hypertension. Small artery in primary pulmonary hypertension in which the lumen is completely occluded by fibrous tissue containing many small vessels. These changes fall in grade 5/6 of the Heath and Edwards classification of pulmonary vascular response to pulmonary hypertension. x350 Hematoxylin and eosin.

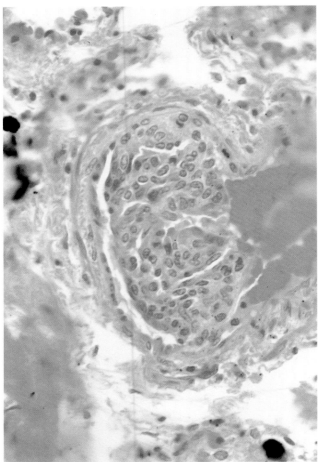

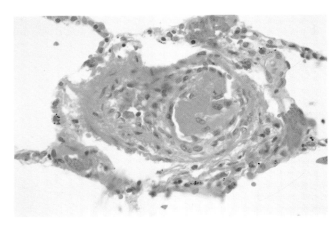

8.11 Thrombo-embolic pulmonary hypertension

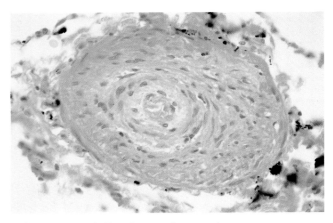

8.10 Vascular changes: pulmonary hypertension

8.12 Thrombo-embolic pulmonary hypertension

8.10 Vascular changes in severe pulmonary hypertension. Small artery in primary pulmonary hypertension where the lumen is partially occluded by a mass of small cuboidal cells with a sinusoidal blood supply. This is a grade 6 change, sometimes called an angiomatoid lesion.
x450 Hematoxylin and eosin.

8.11 Thrombo-embolic pulmonary hypertension. A small pulmonary artery is partially occluded by connective tissue, superimposed on which is a red-staining mass of fibrin.
x275 Hematoxylin and eosin.

8.12 Thrombo-embolic pulmonary hypertension. A small artery from the same case as shown in **8.11**. The vessel lumen is virtually occluded by concentric layers of intimal connective tissue and smooth muscle proliferation. No thrombus is present at this site. No specific histological feature can be used to differentiate thrombo-embolic from primary pulmonary hypertension.
x275 Hematoxylin and eosin.

CHAPTER 9

Cardiac Tumours

SECONDARY INVOLVEMENT OF THE HEART (9.1 – 9.10)

Involvement of the heart and/or pericardium by malignant tumours arising elsewhere is commonplace, whereas primary cardiac tumours are rare. The incidence of cardiac metastases at post-mortem reported in the literature, varies widely. This variation depends on two factors: first, that certain primary sites are more prone than others to involve the heart; thus, any autopsy series which has a high proportion of cases of carcinoma of the bronchus will have a high incidence of cardiac involvement. Secondly, the more histological blocks that are taken of the myocardium at autopsy, the greater will be the number of small myocardial deposits discovered.

The tumours which have a high incidence of cardiac involvement include carcinoma of the bronchus and breast and disseminated malignant melanoma. In these instances cardiac metastases can be found in the heart at autopsy in up to 40% of cases. By contrast, carcinoma of the colon, squamous tumours of tongue or lip, and bladder tumours rarely involve the heart. 'League tables' of the potential for cardiac metastases from individual primary sites of tumour origin are extensively published. Apparent isolated metastases to the heart, sometimes after a long latent period from excision of the primary, are recorded as case reports for virtually every primary site.

Pericardial deposits may occur as multiple nodules or be a diffuse sheet of tumour. In the first instance, large pericardial effusions, often with extensive fibrin deposition over the heart, may be produced. Occasionally the number of tumour cells is small in relation to the degree of acute pericarditis. Myocardial deposits may be multiple or single, and range in size from microscopic foci up to those many centimetres across. Tumour deposits may be entirely confined within the myocardium or bulge externally beneath the pericardium or inward to form a polypoidal mass within a chamber.

The striking clinical feature of secondary carcinoma involving the heart is the great rarity with which clinical symptoms of significance are produced. The only serious sequelae are:

i) production of a tense pericardial effusion or constriction of the heart by solid sheets of tumour;

ii) hemopericardium arising from the surface of a tumour projecting into the pericardial space or rarely following myocardial rupture, particularly of the atria;

iii) emboli arising from intracavity tumour masses, and

iv) obstruction of vessels, particularly the venae cavae or pulmonary veins, by tumours growing within the vessel lumen.

PRIMARY BENIGN CARDIAC TUMOURS (9.11 – 9.21)

All are rare, the commonest being the atrial myxoma. This tumour with few exceptions arises from the limbus of the fossa ovalis. Most examples project into the cavity of the left atrium but an occasional tumour projects into the right atrium and even more rarely a bilobed tumour projects into both atria. The myxoma varies widely in external appearances: some are smooth, and round, others have a multi-fronded papillary appearance. The colour ranges from pale yellow to dark red. The histological appearance, however, is consistent. There is a pale amorphous stroma in which are embedded clumps, cords and gland-like masses of so-called 'lepidic' cells, the name implying a fanciful resemblance to the scales on butterfly wings. The stroma contains abundant connective tissue mucin but very little connective tissue. Deposits of iron, a mixture of inflammatory cells including plasma cells and eosinophils and iron encrusted elastic fragments are very common. Deposits of thrombus are also common, particularly on the surface. Papillary examples are often covered by an external layer of cells resembling those deeper in the stroma. Myxomas are attached by a narrow pedicle to the superficial endocardium from which thick-walled vessels enter the tumour. Tumour cells are never found beneath the endocardium surface.

The clinical presentation of atrial myxomas is variable and diagnosis is often made late. The symptoms fall into two groups: embolic manifestations, and mitral valve obstruction or regurgitation leading to pulmonary hypertension and heart failure. The fronded papillary form of myxoma is particularly liable to present as sudden tumour emboli to the lower limb, retina or brain in an apparently fit individual. All arterial emboli removed at peripheral vascular surgery should be examined histologically to exclude their origin from a myxoma. The more solid tumour leads to mitral valve obstruction or mitral regurgitation. The latter results from a 'wrecking-ball' action of the tumour crossing and recrossing the mitral valve, leading to chordal rupture. Patients with either presentation may have systemic manifestations which include fever, an elevated ESR and hypergammaglobulinemia.

Tumours with the typical histological appearance of an atrial myxoma occasionally arise in the right and left ventricles but are still sufficiently rare to justify individual case reports. The histogenesis of the atrial myxoma is currently linked to cell nests of an 'endothelial-like' or undifferentiated mesenchymal cell sequestered in the formation of the foramen ovale. Atrial myxomata have no potential for malignancy and do not grow even when fragments embolize to the lung. The tumour will, however, recur at the site of atrial excision unless the surgeon actually removes a cuff of muscle or diathermizes around the tumour base.

PRIMARY MALIGNANT CARDIAC TUMOURS (9.22 – 9.29)

The most common cardiac sarcoma is angiomatous in origin, occurring most frequently in the atrium, particularly the right but rapidly spreading to form pericardial and other intracardiac deposits. Tumour may erode into the pericardium producing hemorrhage and tamponade, or grow into the cavity of a chamber. In this instance multiple polypoidal vascular masses of tumour may form, often extending out into the pulmonary artery. Lung metastases or hemopericardium are the usual cause of death.

Rhabdomyosarcomas, myxosarcomas, fibrosarcomas, leiomyosarcomas, and even pure osteogenic sarcomas are all described and usually occur as intracavity polypoidal masses, particularly in the atria and outflow tract of the right ventricle. Many cardiac sarcomas cannot, in practice, be clearly identified as having any particular histogenesis or differentiation. Only if a section shows a vascular differentiation or if tumour cells with cross-striations are found, can the histogenesis be established with certainty. Most case-reports of cardiac sarcomas record the rare instances where there is widespread differentiation along one particular line; most sarcomas encountered in practice are of indeterminate or mixed origin. The macroscopic appearances of these true sarcomas can closely mimic a myxoma although no histological similarity is present. Tumours described as myxosarcomas bear no relation to benign atrial myxomas.

RARE CARDIAC TUMOUR-LIKE MALFORMATIONS (9.30 – 9.41)

Isolated intramyocardial fibromyomata occur, with a macroscopic appearance on their cut surface akin to uterine fibroids. They may be encountered in infancy when large enough to cause death, but more commonly they are coincidental findings in adult autopsies. Multiple intramyocardial nodules usually described as rhabdomyomata occur in tuberose sclerosis and are composed of clear vacuolated cells often compared to the Purkinje cells of the conduction system. The mesothelioma of the atrioventricular node is a small cystic mass up to 2cm across,

occurring in the right atrium immediately anterior to the coronary sinus. Nodal destruction leads to sudden death and or heart block. True teratomatous lesions with all tissue elements present are also described.

Intra-cardiac lipomas, usually appearing as sub-endocardial yellow lobulated masses, are small and coincidental findings at autopsy. They must be distinguished from the extensive infiltration between muscle fibres by fatty tissue that is found in most hearts from old people. Benign hemangiomas project from the pericardial surface of the atria and are also coincidental autopsy findings.

Small papillary masses, often with a sessile base and having a fanciful similarity to viral warts of the skin, occur on the endocardial surface of the mitral and aortic valves. While their histological appearance has been likened to atrial myxomata, this similarity is simply fortuitous and they are most likely to represent organization of small thrombi over years. Known as myxo-papillary tumours of valve, they are rarely of any clinical significance. Their significance is perhaps greatest in the confusion they create in surgeons, echocardiographers and pathologists on their first encounter with the lesion. Their incidence is highest on abnormal valves; in very rare instances small emboli arise from their surface.

Pericardial cysts may occur as coincidental findings on chest X-ray, echocardiography or autopsy. They are thin-walled cysts attached to the visceral surface of the pericardium, usually over the ventricles. The contents may be clear fluid or inspissated mucus. The lining epithelium is either mesothelial or more frequently columnar, suggesting gastrointestinal mucosa.

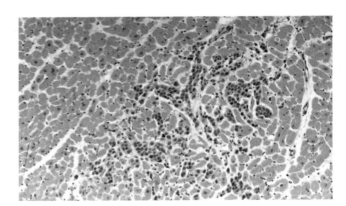

9.1 Metastatic tumour

9.1 Myocardial metastatic tumour. Histological section of the left ventricle in a woman dying of metastatic breast carcinoma. No cardiac symptoms were noted. No macroscopic abnormality of the heart was noted but routine histological examination showed this small focus of carcinoma in the interstitial tissue of the myocardium. x45 Hematoxylin and eosin.

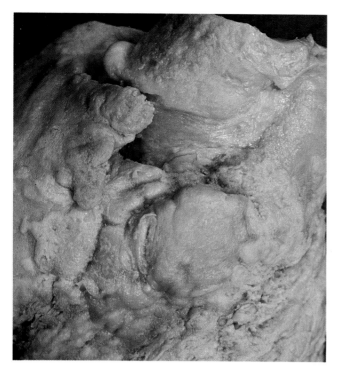

9.2 Pericardial metastatic tumour

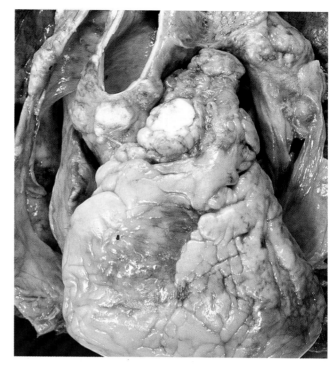

9.3 Pericardial metastatic tumour

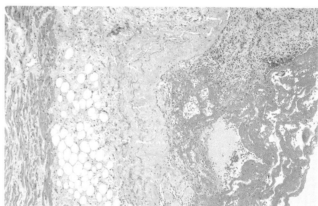

9.4 Pericardial metastatic tumour

9.2   Pericardial secondary tumour. Diffuse sheets of tumour cover the visceral pericardium of the heart in a patient with carcinoma of the bronchus. Tumour deposits of this type may lead to pericardial constriction. Tumour may reach the pericardium by direct spread or via lymphatics.

9.3   Pericardial secondary tumour. The visceral pericardium shows nodules of a white tumour over the base of the aorta and atrium. Such deposits are often asymptomatic; rarely, they lead to large blood-stained diffusions.

9.4   Pericardial secondary tumour. Extensive deposits of red-staining fibrin on the pericardium, undergoing early organization, in a patient with carcinoma of the breast. The adipose tissue beneath the pericardium and the underlying myocardium show infiltration by acute and chronic inflammatory cells, but tumour cells are not present.
x300 Hematoxylin and eosin.

9.5   Pericardial secondary tumour. An area adjacent to that shown in **9.4**. The pericardium shows proliferation of small blood vessels and an acute and chronic inflammatory cell infiltrate but in addition islands of tumour cells are apparent. The fibrinous response in this area is slight.
x100 Hematoxylin and eosin.

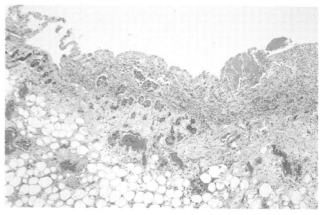

9.5 Pericardial metastatic tumour

9.6 Multiple intramyocardial secondary deposits.
Multiple pigmented intramyocardial deposits are evenly distributed in the left ventricular myocardium of a patient with disseminated malignant melanoma. It is reputed that the heart of Catharine of Aragon showed such an appearance.

9.7 Secondary carcinoma of the heart. A short axis view of the myocardium shows all three features of secondary carcinoma that can be recognized by echocardiography. The tumour involves the posterior wall of the left ventricle. It has an intramyocardial component, a component which bulges beneath the pericardium and a component which has eroded into the cavity of the right ventricle (arrows) to form a polypoidal mass covered by thrombus. The primary site was the urinary bladder.

9.8 Secondary carcinoma of the heart. Long axis view of the heart showing an isolated secondary deposit from a carcinoma of the kidney in the interventricular septal myocardium which does not involve the cavity of the ventricle. The septal thickening produced by such a deposit may simulate hypertrophic cardiomyopathy.

9.9 Secondary carcinoma involving the vena cava.
Tumour projecting into the right atrium from the inferior vena cava which is totally occluded by a tumour which was in direct continuity with a malignant hepatoma of the liver. Propagation of the tumour along the venae cavae is a feature of renal adenocarcinoma, hepatocellular carcinomas, and carcinoma of the bronchus. Malignant tumours of the lung may also extend along pulmonary veins to form a mass in the left atrium.

9.10 Secondary carcinoma involving the right atrium. The heart has been opened to show the interatrial septum viewed from the right. In the orifice of the inferior vena cava and covering the coronary sinus and foramen ovale is a lobulated round tumour. This lesion was initially diagnosed by echocardiography as a right atrial myxoma. Subsequent investigation showed this tumour to extend all along the vena cava from a primary carcinoma of the. kidney.

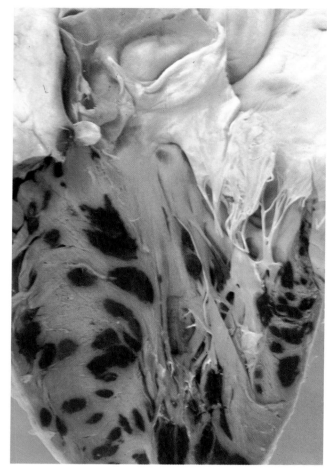

9.6 Intramyocardial metastatic deposits

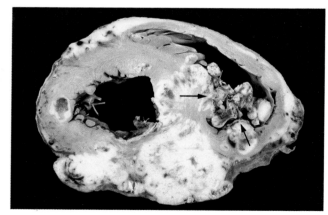

9.7 Metastatic carcinoma

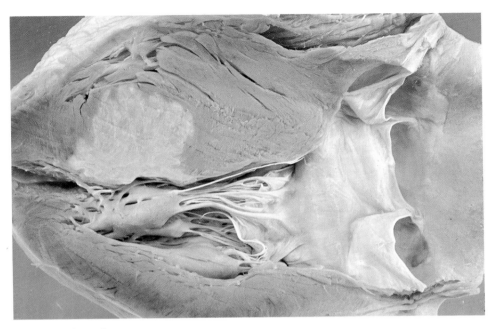

9.8 Metastatic carcinoma

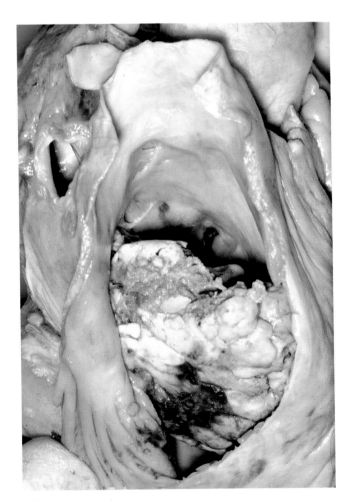

9.9 Metastatic carcinoma: vena cava

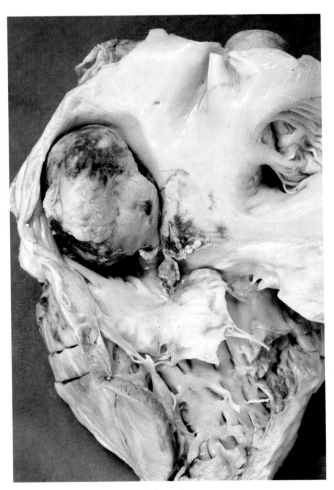

9.10 Metastatic carcinoma: right atrium

9.11 Left atrial myxoma. Left atrial myxoma surgically-excised and fixed in formalin. This is the usual appearance of such a specimen, showing a partially-lobulated yellow tumour with a mostly smooth surface but showing some wrinkling with areas of darker red hemorrhage and thrombus deposition on the surface.

9.12 Left atrial myxoma. Surgically-excised left atrial myxoma in the fresh state prior to fixation. The tumour is a glistening, smooth, rounded mass without the rather wrinkled appearance that develops after fixation. Many have the yellow-red colour shown here. A small cuff of endocardium (arrows) marks the site of attachment to the foramen ovale, and myxomas can always be shelled out in this way. Little force is needed. Very occasionally the tumour spontaneously avulses to lie free in the atrium.

9.13 Left atrial myxoma. A small atrial myxoma attached to the fossa ovalis viewed from above, in the left atrium looking down on the mitral valve. The tumour is very dark, from the presence of much surface thrombosis.

Death was due to a large cerebral embolus and the myxoma was previously asymptomatic. The embolus in this case was largely thrombotic rather than tumour fragments.

9.14 Left atrial myxoma. Both atria are viewed from above, looking down on the mitral and tricuspid valves. A large left atrial myxoma is present, which had almost totally occluded the mitral orifice, leading to cardiac failure. This tumour is a large round mass which was very soft and yellow at post-mortem and attached by a tiny pedicle to the fossa ovalis. A ridge marked the junction between the upper mass of tumour in the atria and a lower portion which was impacting into the mitral valve orifice.

9.15 Left atrial myxoma. A large left atrial myxoma attached to the left side of the fossa ovalis and protruding down into the mitral valve orifice. This tumour had a broad base and a very villous papillary surface. This papillary type of myxoma has a high risk of producing tumour emboli.

Reference:

McAllister H A and Genoglio J J. Tumours of the Cardiovascular System. Washington D C: Armed Forces Institute of Pathology 1977.

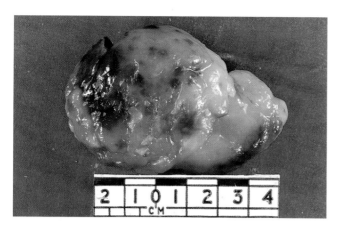

9.11 Atrial myxoma

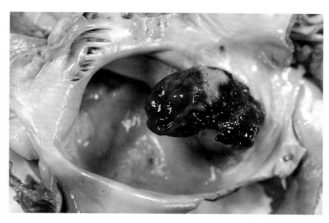

9.13 Atrial myxoma

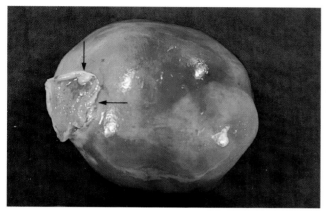

9.12 Atrial myxoma

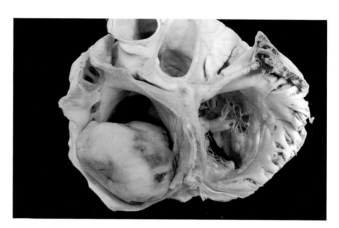

9.14 Atrial myxoma

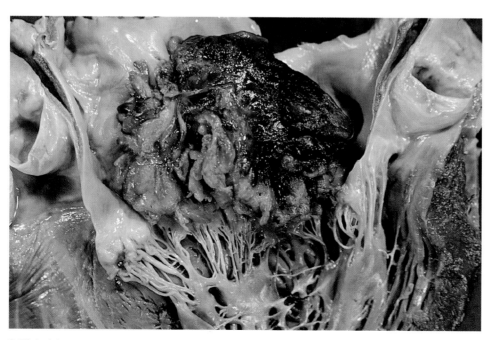

9.15 Atrial myxoma

9.16 Right atrial myxoma. The right atrium has been opened to show the right side of the atrial septum. The tumour is a round white smooth mass attached to the foramen ovale by a stalk (arrow). This stalk allowed the tumour to prolapse into the tricuspid valve orifice. The myxoma was heavily calcified and the patient's age, 78, suggested that it had been present for many years. The surface was smooth and covered by endothelium, and had no surface thrombus.

9.17 Right atrial myxoma. This tumour is a smooth round dark mass attached to the foramen ovale. The tumour had a high proportion of incorporated surface thrombus and it is easy to misinterpret such a lesion as a simple ball thrombus. Some specimens of atrial ball thrombi on display in pathology museums are in fact atrial myxomas.

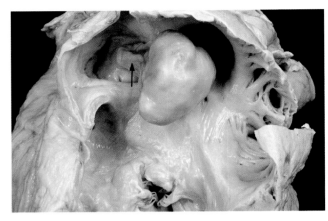

9.16 Right atrial myxoma

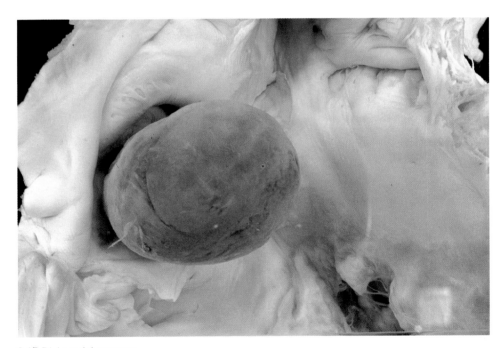

9.17 Right atrial myxoma

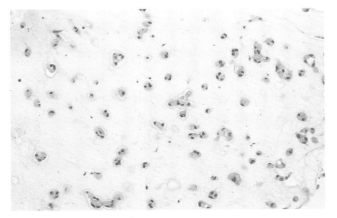

9.18 Atrial myxoma

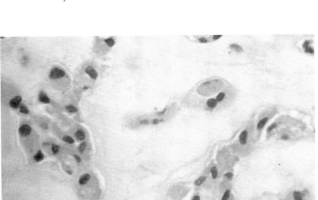

9.19 Atrial myxoma

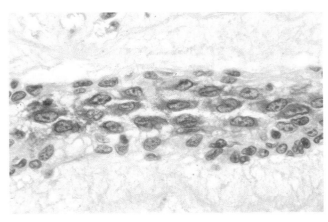

9.20 Atrial myxoma

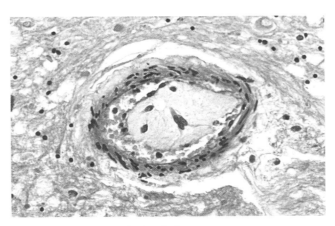

9.21 Atrial myxoma: cerebral emboli

9.18   Atrial myxoma: histology. Histological section of an atrial myxoma showing a basophilic stroma within which are embedded cords and nests of cells. In many cases iron- and calcium-impregnated fibrils are present in the stroma as well as hemosiderin granules.
x100 Hematoxylin and eosin.

9.19   Atrial myxoma: histology. Higher-power view of the so-called lepidic (scale-like) cells of a myxoma. The cells have eosinophilic cytoplasm and small dark nuclei. They are arranged in clumps or threads often around a central space.
x300 Hematoxylin and eosin.

9.20   Atrial myxoma: cell origin. Groups of 'lepidic' cells in an atrial myxoma stained for Factor VIII-related antigen by the immunoperoxidase technique. The cells contain brown-red granules indicating the presence of the antigen and by implication the endothelial origin of the 'myxoma'. Positive staining is usually present in the centre of clumps of cells, rather than in single cells in the stroma.
x450 Immunoperoxidase for Factor VIII.

9.21   Atrial myxoma: cerebral emboli. Histological section of the brain from a patient with a left atrial myxoma. A small artery is totally occluded by a fragment of myxoma without associated thrombus formation. One month before a retinal embolus occurred followed by massive brain stem infarction leading to death. Previously asymptomatic.
x225 Hematoxylin and eosin.

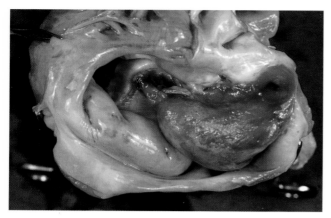

9.22 Angiosarcoma

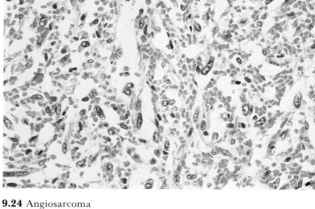

9.24 Angiosarcoma

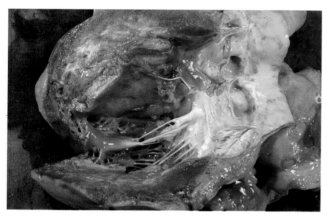

9.23 Angiosarcoma

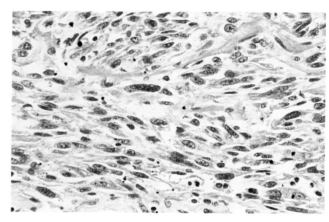

9.25 Angiosarcoma

9.22 Angiosarcoma. Angiosarcoma arising in the left atrium viewed from above looking down on the mitral valve. The tumour is solid and red with a wide base. The macroscopic appearances could easily be mistaken for an atrial myxoma or for simple mural thrombus and the diagnosis was only made easy by the presence of tumour nodules in the other chambers.

9.23 Angiosarcoma. Angiosarcoma in the left ventricle. Tumour invades the ventricular septum and has led to massive overlying thrombus formation. Histological sections of deeper parts of the lesion must be taken for diagnostic purposes, because superficial zones of angiosarcomas are usually totally necrotic or merely thrombus, making biopsies taken in life very unreliable for diagnosis.

9.24 Angiosarcoma: histology. Histological section of an angiosarcoma of the heart from an area which has good histological differentiation and vascular spaces containing red cells. While vascular spaces are present the nuclei of the lining cells are very large, unlike a benign angioma. x200 Hematoxylin and eosin.

9.25 Angiosarcoma: histology. Another area of the angiosarcoma of the heart shown in **9.24**. Here the tumour is solid, with numerous elongated fusiform cells, very bizarre nuclei, and numerous mitoses. Many of the cells have eosinophilic cytoplasm and are indistinguishable from those seen in tumours designated as rhabdomyosarcomas, except that cross-striations are absent. Small biopsies of intracavitary sarcomas, but particularly those of angiomatomas types, may only obtain thrombus from the surface or well-differentiated areas, and the true nature of the tumour is masked.
x275 Hematoxylin and eosin.

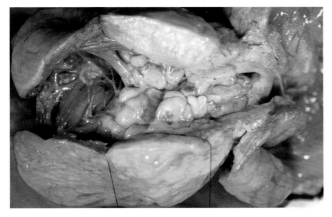

9.26 Primary sarcoma

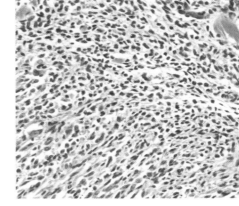

9.28 Sarcoma of the heart

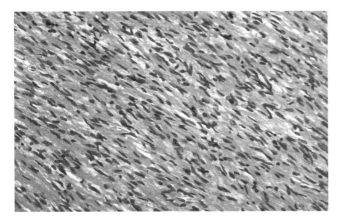

9.27 Sarcoma of the heart

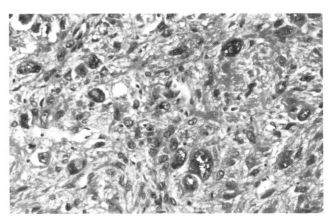

9.29 Sarcoma of the heart

9.26 Primary sarcoma of the heart. The outflow tract of the right ventricle has been opened through the pulmonary valve into the pulmonary artery. The wall of the right ventricular outflow (infundibular area) is totally replaced by a thick layer of white tumour. Tumour extends into the cavity as a lobulated mass which has grown up the outflow tract destroying the pulmonary valve. This mode of spread is common to all forms of sarcoma involving the right side of the heart, and it is also adopted by some secondary tumours. Clinically, obstruction to right heart outflow is produced. Echo and angiographic diagnosis of a mass moving in the pulmonary artery is straightforward. Death usually results from pulmonary emboli of tumour or thrombus.

9.27 Sarcoma of the heart: histology. Multiple lobulated nodules of tumour were found in the right ventricular outflow, extending through the pulmonary valve and invading the pulmonary artery wall. Death followed a surgical attempt to resect the tumour, which is a sarcoma with densely-packed, parallel arranged, spindle-shaped cells. Special stains demonstrated the presence of both connective tissue and smooth muscle. The histogenesis is arguably that of fibrosarcoma or leiomyosarcoma.
x175 Hematoxylin and eosin.

9.28 Sarcoma of the heart: histology. Histological section from a lobulated intramyocardial tumour which projected into the apices of both ventricular cavities. The tumour is composed of loosely and irregularly arranged spindle cells with a considerable number of lymphocytes and plasma cells at the margin where residual myocardial cells are present. The histogenesis is not apparent in this field.
x175 Hematoxylin and eosin.

9.29 Sarcoma of the heart: histology. Higher-power view of part of **9.28**. In this particular field tumour giant cells with large bizarre nuclei are present. The appearances suggest that this sarcoma is of cardiac muscle origin but no cross-striations could be shown by conventional methods. The patient died of multiple lung metastases within a few months of presentation.
x250 Hematoxylin and eosin.

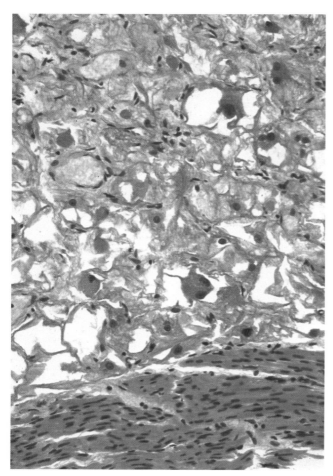

9.30 Tuberose sclerosis

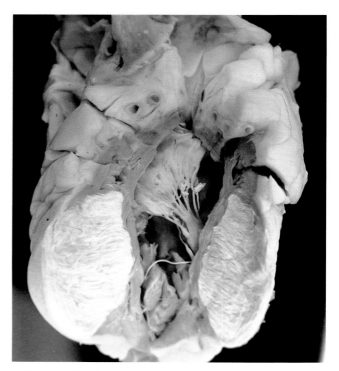

9.31 Myocardial fibroma

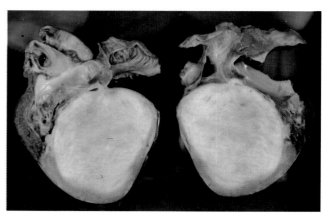

9.32 Myocardial fibroma

9.30   Tuberose sclerosis: myoma of myocardium.
Section from a nodule in the myocardium of a patient
known to have tuberose sclerosis. The nodule is composed
of vacuolated cells which have peripheral myofibrils and
are far larger than the adjacent normal myocardial cells
(M). It is the clear cytoplasm of these cells that is likened
to the normal Purkinje cell.
x350 Hematoxylin and eosin.

9.31   Myocardial fibroma. The lateral wall of the left
ventricle has been opened to show that the tumour is
well-demarcated, white and solid, with a whorled cut
surface. Coincidental finding at autopsy in an accidental
death.

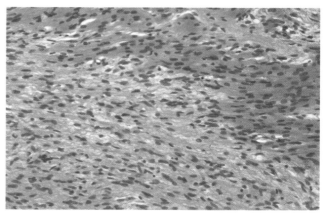

9.33 Myocardial fibroma

9.32 Infantile myocardial fibroma. The heart is from an infant who had a large septal tumour obstructing the outflow of the left ventricle, producing heart block and leading to sudden death. The heart has been bisected to show a massive white tumour in the ventricular septum.

9.33 Myocardial fibroma: histology. Myocardial fibromyomata in a child. The tumour is a complex mixture of connective tissue, smooth muscle and residual islands of myocardial muscle cells. No cell pleomorphism is present. The tumour is regarded as fibroma or fibromyoma and is totally benign.
x150 Hematoxylin and eosin.

9.34 Mesothelioma of atrioventricular node. Section across the area of the atrioventricular node in a young patient who died suddenly and in whom a cystic nodule 1cm in diameter was present, just beneath the right atrial endocardium anterior to the coronary sinus. The A-V node should be between the central fibrous body (CFB) and right atrial (RA) endocardium: in this area, however, there are multiple cystic spaces and no nodal tissue can be seen.
x25 Hematoxylin and eosin.

9.35 Mesothelioma of atrioventricular node. Higher-power view of the nodal area shown in **9.34**. The node is replaced by cystic spaces lined by epithelium and containing eosinophilic material. Some cysts are apparently empty, others contain more solid nests of cells. The cells lining the cysts may be squamoid, columnar or flattened. The intra-cystic material proved to be PAS-positive.
x95 Hematoxylin and eosin.

9.36 Mesothelioma of atrioventricular node. Mesothelioma of atrioventricular node in which the cysts are lined by flattened epithelium and contain oval 'bodies'. Solid nests of epithelial cells are also present in the fibrous stroma. The very much rarer true teratoma of the heart contains identifiable cartilage, columnar mucus secreting epithelium as well as neural tissue. The mesothelioma is regarded as arising from pericardial tissue sequestered in the nodal area.
x95 Hematoxylin and eosin.

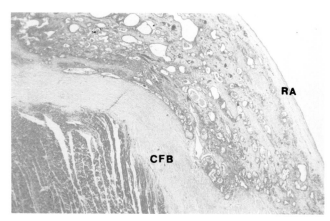

9.34 Mesothelioma

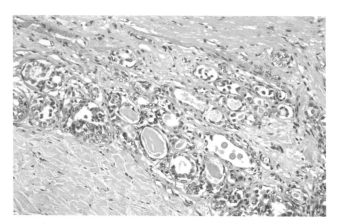

9.35 Mesothelioma

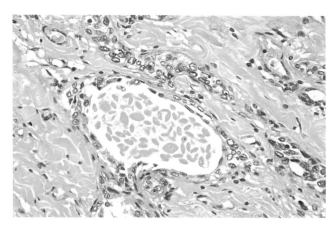

9.36 Mesothelioma

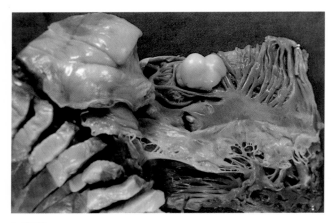

9.37 Lipoma

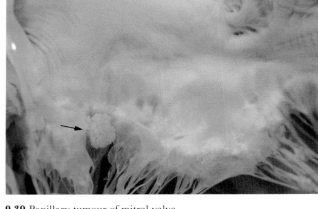

9.39 Papillary tumour of mitral valve

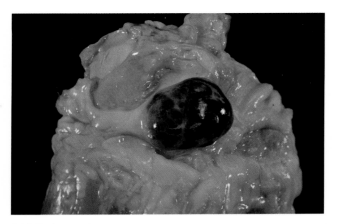

9.38 Benign angioma

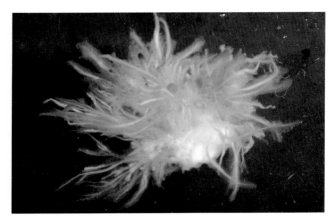

9.40 Papillary tumour

9.37 Lipoma of the heart. A small subendocardial lipoma is present in the right atrium or projects into the cavity. Lipomas are incidental autopsy findings.

9.38 Benign angioma. The posterior pericardial surface of the heart contains a blood-filled mass 3cm across. Angiomas may reach a vast size and have a rich blood flow, making their angiographic confirmation an easy task in life. They are usually discovered at examination in life or as coincidental autopsy findings.

9.39 Papillary tumour of mitral valve. The tumour (arrow) has a sessile base and a papillary surface. The valve is otherwise normal.

9.40 Papillary tumour of cardiac valve. The tumour is viewed under water by dissecting microscopy. The papillary and fronded structure of the tumour is well demonstrated in this way. These myxopapillary lesions of valve cusps are neither true tumours nor related to atrial myxoma.

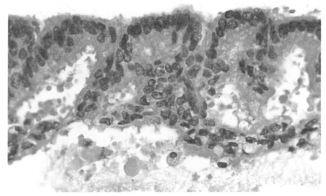

9.41 Pericardial cyst

9.41 Pericardial cyst of the heart. The cyst was attached to the apex of the left ventricle and was seen on chest X-ray and explored surgically. The lining is columnar and thrown in folds beneath which there are glandular structures. Some of the surface cells are ciliated. This appearance is the most typical of simple cysts although the exact histogenesis is arguable.
x600 Hematoxylin and eosin.

CHAPTER 10

Congenital Heart Disease

Ninety per cent of congenital heart disease falls into two categories, being either defects involving 'holes' with shunts between chambers, or obstructing lesions to valve orifices or aorta. The remainder, a small minority, are highly complex defects with an infinite variety of types. Only the former and larger group is considered here. The latter are the preserve of specialized texts on congenital heart disease. At this simple level, a functional classification of congenital heart disease can be made into: (a) those which initially shunt blood from left to right and are not associated with cyanosis; (b) those shunting blood from right to left and associated with cyanosis; and (c) purely obstructive lesions.

LEFT-TO-RIGHT SHUNTS (10.1 – 10.18)

The group of conditions which produce non-cyanotic left-to-right shunts include the atrial septal defects, ventricular septal defects, and patent ductus arteriosus. All are associated with an increase in pulmonary blood flow due to the shunt and thus initially lead to right ventricular volume overload. Later, as pulmonary artery pressures rise, the right ventricle is subjected to pressure overload. The clinical features and natural history of the three conditions differ, however, in many aspects.

A persistently patent ductus arteriosus is simply a retention of the fetal structure which *in utero* by-passes the lungs. The ductus joins the main pulmonary artery, of which it is a continuation, directly to the aorta, and it may be of the same internal calibre as these structures. A patent duct can usually be recognized both by its loud murmur and the fact that it produces early cardiac failure. Distinction must be made between prolonged or delayed closure of a duct in a small or premature infant, in whom closure will occur with time or encouragement by indomethacin, and true patent ductus. In the latter the internal elastic lamina persists in the duct which also fails to develop the usual medial muscular hyperplasia.

Atrial septal defects fall into several categories. The most common is the so-called ostium secundum defect which arises at the site of the foramen ovale. When the fibrous floor of the foramen ovale is deficient, a septal defect results. In the largest secundum defects the posterior rim of the fossa ovalis is absent and the posterior atrial wall forms the margin of the defect. All secundum defects, however, have atrial septal tissue separating their inferior margins from the tricuspid valve.

The flow from left to right across the defect is not strictly a result of pressure difference. It arises from the relative ease with which the right ventricle fills as compared to the left. No murmur is generated at the site of the shunt and the physical signs are a subtle blend of a systolic pulmonary flow murmur and delayed closure of the pulmonary valve. Diagnosis is thus not often made until adolescence or later. In association with secundum atrial septal defects, there are a number of mitral valve abnormalities. Classically, an association of rheumatic disease and an atrial septal defect is Lutembacher's syndrome. In retrospect the condition was never perhaps very common but led to a collection of physical signs which clinicians found fascinating. Most secundum defects are found to have very specific but ill-understood secondary changes in the medial half of the anterior cusp of the mitral valve, but these are of minimal functional significance. A small proportion of patients with secundum atrial defects do develop mitral regurgitation, now thought to be related to an associated under-development of the posterior cusp of the mitral valve.

The ostium primum type of atrial septal defect lies inferior to the foramen ovale. The condition is part of a spectrum of complex changes described as the persistent common atrioventricular canal or endocardial cushion defects. The atrial component of this spectrum is a defect with a crescentic upper border formed by the foramen ovale and without any atrial septal tissue on its inferior border, which is formed by tricuspid valve tissue. A purely atrial defect, without any abnormality of the atrioventricular valves, is one extreme of the spectrum. Most ostium primum defects have associated abnormalities of the atrioventricular valves, particularly a deep cleft in the anterior cusp of the mitral valve. In the complete type of persistent common atrioventricular canal, an atrial septal defect is combined with a ventricular septal defect, and one atrioventricular valve is common to both ventricles passing through the defect. This lesion is a common form of congenital heart disease in Down's syndrome (mongolism).

Sinus venosus-type atrial septal defects lie superior to the fossa ovalis close to the superior atrial junction, and are associated with anomalous termination of one or more of the right-sided pulmonary veins.

Ventricular septal defects are usually divided into the common form, occurring in the region of the membranous interventricular septum just below the aortic valve, and the much rarer defect in the muscular septum. The membranous defects are actually far more complex than simple failure of the membranous septum and usually they also involve portions of the inlet, outlet and trabecular inter-ventricular muscular septum. They can be further sub-divided by their relation to the crista supraventricularis and papillary muscle of the conus.

Ventricular septal defects vary widely in their clinical manifestations but many can be suspected early in life from the murmur they generate from the high pressure turbulent flow through the defect. The development of symptoms depends on the size of the defects. Defects smaller in area than the aortic valve create a very loud murmur but little hemodynamic effect, and the patient is asymptomatic. Larger defects precipitate left ventricular failure early in life. Spontaneous closure of ventricular septal defects can occur, both by growth of the muscular septum and by adhesions of the tricuspid valve leaflets to the edges of the defect.

All of the left-to-right shunt situations can be com-plicated by, first, the development of labile pulmonary hypertension followed subsequently by rising pressures which ultimately exceed systemic levels and allow shunt reversal with the appearances of cyanosis (Eisenmenger's syndrome). In both large ventricular septal defects and widely patent ductus arteriosus, the Eisenmenger syn-drome can develop early in childhood and is associated with striking morphological changes in the pulmonary vessels. Where the pulmonary pressure has been at systemic level from birth, the media of the main pul-monary arteries retain an elastic pattern more reminiscent of the aortic media. The initial phase of the disease is associated with striking medial hypertrophy in the muscular arteries and proximal arterioles. As irreversible pulmonary hypertension develops, the intima becomes fibrous, and finally plexiform and angiomatoid lesions form. Patients with atrial septal defects do not usually develop shunt reversal until late in adult life, and the onset of irreversible pulmonary hypertension is often related to the development of small pulmonary emboli.

Bacterial endocarditis is a risk in all situations with a high pressure flow and thus complicates patent ductus and ventricular septal defects, but not secundum atrial septal defects. Ostium primum septal defects are at risk from the abnormal mitral valve.

CYANOTIC CONGENITAL HEART DISEASE RIGHT-TO-LEFT SHUNTS
(10.19 – 10.25)

The two relatively common forms of congenital heart disease that cause cyanosis from birth are Fallot's tetra-logy and complete transposition of the great vessels. Fallot's tetralogy is a combination of obstruction to pul-monary flow due to hypoplasia and dysplasia of the right ventricular outflow, with a ventricular septal defect. The remaining two facets of the tetralogy can be deduced and are an apparent shift and enlargement of the aortic outflow (overriding or straddling the aorta) due to the small pul-monary outflow and secondary right ventricular hyper-

trophy. The right ventricular outflow obstruction can be any combination of pulmonary artery atresia or hypo-plasia, valve stenosis and infundibular obstruction, and varies markedly from case to case. The ventricular septal defect is in the membranous septal area, but often has no muscle rim under the aortic valve. Patients with Fallot's tetralogy develop cyanosis with the consequence of poly-cythemia and venous thrombus which may invoke para-doxical emboli.

Complete transposition of the great vessels is simply a reversal of the aortic and pulmonary outflows. The aorta opens from the right ventricle. A free communication at either or both atrial and ventricular levels is essential to allow pulmonary/systemic blood mixing and survival.

OBSTRUCTIVE CONGENITAL HEART DISEASE
(10.26 – 10.29)

The two common forms of obstructive congenital heart disease are isolated pulmonary valve stenosis and coarc-tation of the aorta. In isolated pulmonary stenosis, the valve is a dome with a central orifice without formed cusps. Valvotomy in early life is highly successful. If untreated, a massive right ventricle develops which can further lead to infundibular stenosis secondary to the muscular hypertrophy.

The common form of coarctation of the aorta is a localized fibrous stricture close to the site of the ductus. The aorta proximal to the obstruction dilates and may rupture spontaneously. Collateral flow develops via numerous arteries, particularly the subcostal and internal mammary arteries. Bicuspid aortic valves are a common association. In tubular hypoplasia of the aorta, a segment, usually between the left subclavian artery and the ductus, is uniformly narrowed. This is usually associated with a patent ductus and often other congenital cardiac abnorm-alities.

CONGENITAL ABNORMALITIES OF CORONARY ARTERIES
(10.30 – 10.33)

There is an infinite variation in the anatomy of the distal branches of the coronary artery tree and the areas of myocardium which they supply. The inverse relation in size between the left circumflex and right coronary artery is discussed in relation to dominance in Chapter 1.

Some congenital anomalies involve the origin of the coronary arteries from the aorta. The coronary ostia nor-mally arise just above the supra-aortic ridge. They can, however, be found as much as 2cm above the ridge, in the sinus itself or even at a valve commissure. Such ano-malous origins are only important to a clinician attempting angiography. If the right aortic sinus is examined carefully, in 20% of individuals there is found a small third opening, the conus artery supplying the outflow tract of the right ventricle.

A major anomaly is present when the aorta contains only a single coronary artery orifice. This may be the single origin of both main arteries and can be in the right or left sinus. In such cases the artery which has no opening from the sinus arises as a first branch of the other main artery. The right or left artery respectively, therefore, has to cross the front of the heart to reach its normal position. If this crossing is made in front of the pulmonary trunk, the anomaly is clinically safe. If the crossing is between the pulmonary and aortic trunk, the artery undergoes obliteration over some years, potentially leading to infarction.

The other alternative when one orifice is found in the aorta is that the other is in the pulmonary trunk. In this case, blood is shunted through the coronary arteries from left to right. The coronary arteries become tortuous and widely dilated as a result of a large blood flow. The subendocardial zone of the myocardium develops fibrosis and often calcifies.

References:

Anderson R H, Becker A E, Lucchese F E, Meier M A, Rogby M L and Soto B. Morphology of Congenital Heart Disease. Tunbridge Wells: Castle House 1983.

Becker A E and Anderson R H. Pathology of Congenital Heart Disease. London: Butterworths 1981.

Becker A E and Anderson R H. Cardiac Pathology. Edinburgh: Churchill Livingstone 1984.

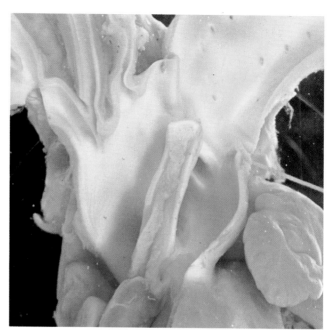

10.1 Patent ductus arteriosus

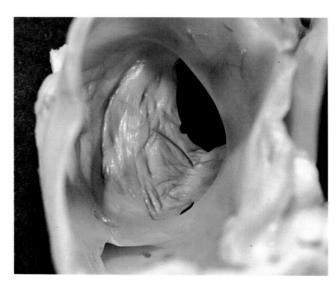

10.2 Atrial septal defect

10.1 Patent ductus arteriosus. Patent ductus arteriosus which appears as a continuation of the main pulmonary artery, and which joins directly into the aorta. In this case the cross-sectional area of the aorta, main pulmonary artery and duct are very similar.

10.2, 10.3 Atrial septal defect. Small secundum atrial septal defect viewed from the right atrium. In **10.2** the defect is a single hole due to partial absence of the floor of the fossa ovalis. In **10.3** the defect is due to fenestration of the floor of the fossa ovalis leading to several holes. The coronary sinus lies below and behind the defects which have clearly defined muscle forming their lower border and separating them from the tricuspid valve.

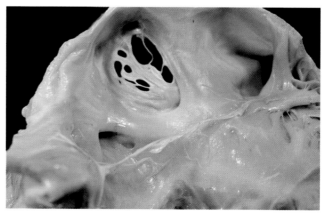

10.3 Atrial septal defect

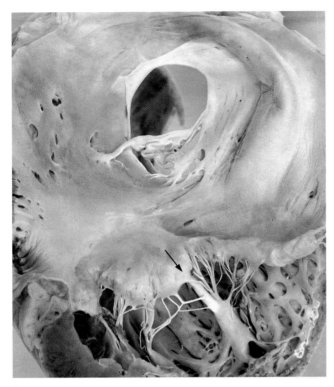

10.4 Atrial septal defect

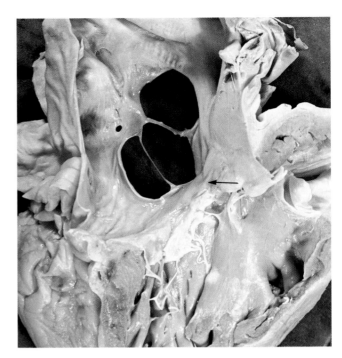

10.5 Atrial septal defect

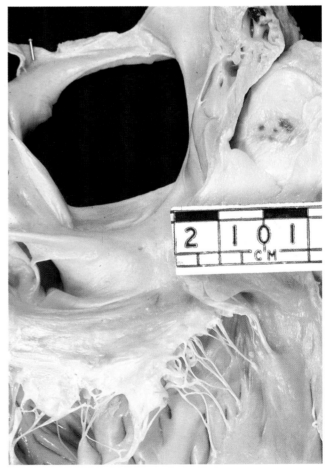

10.6 Atrial septal defect

10.4   Large atrial septal defect. A large secundum atrial septal defect viewed from the left atrium. The mitral valve shows an abnormality almost universally present in hearts with secundum atrial defects, which consists of thickened chordae at the medial commissure and a slightly domed and thickened anterior cusp (arrow). This lesion probably develops as a secondary change to some ill-understood mechanical or flow change. The lower rim of the defect is separated from the mitral valve by a considerable distance, the muscle of the lower atrial septum intervening.

10.5   Large atrial septal defect. A large atrial septal defect viewed from the right atrium. The defect involves the whole foramen ovale which is also deficient on the anterior and the inferior margin. A rim of tissue (arrow), however, just separates the defect from the tricuspid valve whose morphology is normal. This is still a secundum type septal defect although considerably larger than the foramen ovale itself. The foramen ovale is the upper of the three holes.

10.6   Large atrial septal defect. A very large atrial septal defect viewed from the right side. There is virtually no atrial septum. The tricuspid valve, however, is normal, and still well separated from the defect. This form of defect is sometimes functionally known as a common atrium but in fact there are still two atria, and two normal appendages are present.

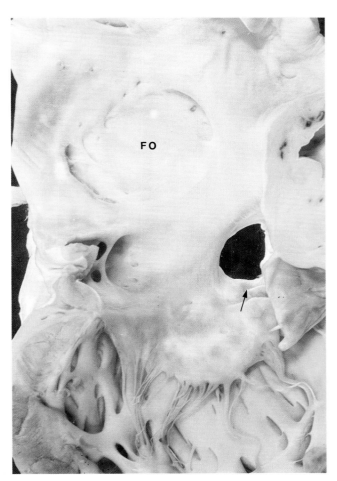

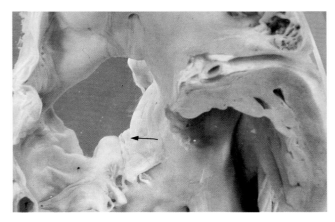

10.8 Primum atrial septal defect

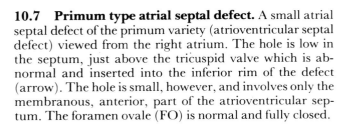

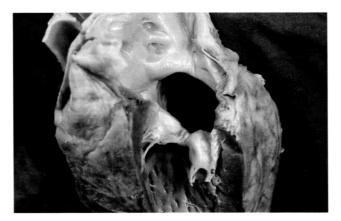

10.7 Primum atrial septal defect

10.9 Primum atrial septal defect

10.7 Primum type atrial septal defect. A small atrial septal defect of the primum variety (atrioventricular septal defect) viewed from the right atrium. The hole is low in the septum, just above the tricuspid valve which is abnormal and inserted into the inferior rim of the defect (arrow). The hole is small, however, and involves only the membranous, anterior, part of the atrioventricular septum. The foramen ovale (FO) is normal and fully closed.

10.8 Primum type atrial septal defect. A large atrial septal defect of the primum (atrioventricular type). The hole involves both the more anterior membranous part of the atrial septum as well as the muscular portion.

Posteriorly, the defect extends almost to the coronary sinus. The tricuspid valve is inserted into the inferior rim of the hole (arrow).

10.9 Atrial septal defect of the primum type. Atrial septal defect of the primum (atrioventricular type) viewed from the left atrium. The defect comes right down to the mitral valve which is itself grossly abnormal. Instead of anterior and posterior cusps there are two 'bridging' leaflets inserted into the lower border of the defect. This leaves an apparent cleft in the anterior cusp which is, however, in reality formed by the gap between the anterior and posterior bridging leaflets.

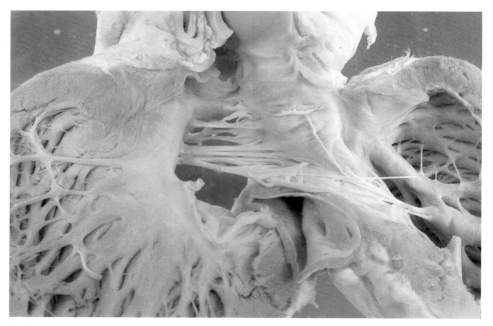

10.10 Atrio-ventricular canal

10.10 Atrio-ventricular canal defect. Common atrioventricular canal viewed from the left ventricle. There is a large ventricular septal defect combined with a primum type atrial septal defect through which a common valve tricuspid and mitral valve bridges left and right atria.

10.11 Ventricular septal defect. Typical peri-membranous ventricular septal defect viewed from the left ventricular outflow. The defect is immediately beneath the aortic valve but there is a rim of tissue on the upper margin (arrow) which does separate the valve and the defect.

10.12 Ventricular septal defect. The same peri-membranous ventricular septal defect as **10.11** viewed from the right ventricle. The defect opens into the right ventricular outflow beneath the crista supraventricularis (CV) and is characteristically tear-drop shaped.

10.13 Ventricular septal defect. A large ventricular septal defect viewed from the left side. The defect is immediately beneath the aortic valve. The red marker shows the tiny ridge which is the main atrioventricular bundles of His lying on the crest of the muscular interventricular septum which forms the lower rim of the defect. At this site the conduction is clearly in danger of being disrupted when a patch is sutured across the defect.

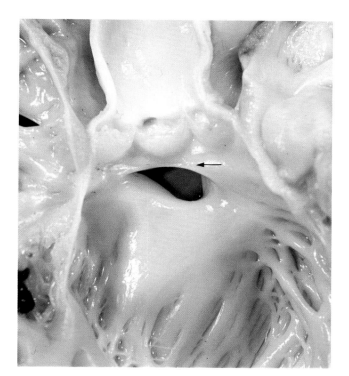

10.11 Ventricular septal defect

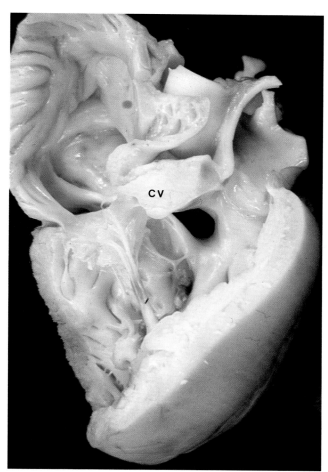

10.12 Ventricular septal defect

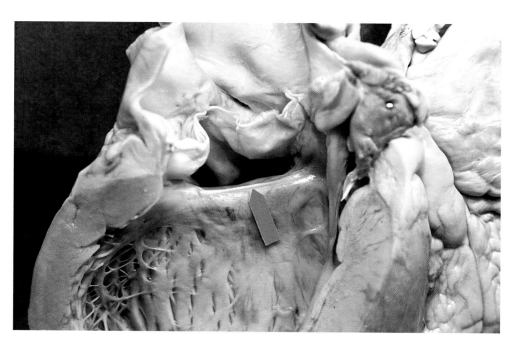

10.13 Ventricular septal defect

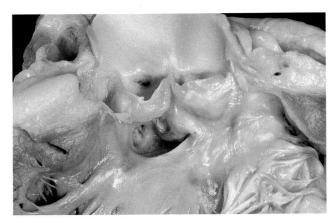

10.14 Aneurysm: membranous septum

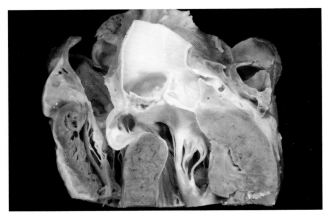

10.15 Aneurysm: membranous septum

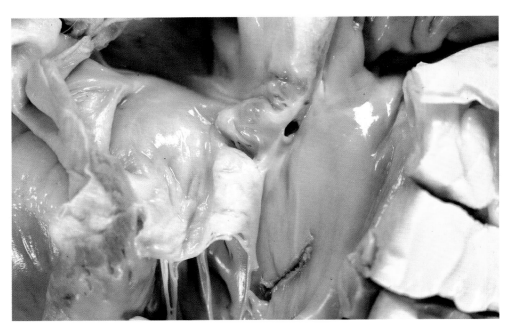

10.16 Self-closing septal defect

10.14 Aneurysm of the membranous ventricular septum. An aneurysm of the membranous interventricular septum, forming a sac just beneath the aortic valve. This is actually a ventricular septal defect which has been closed by tricuspid valve tissue adhering to the rim of the hole. The valve tissue can be seen forming the floor of the aneurysm. The majority of so-called aneurysms in this region are of this type.

10.15 Aneurysm of the membranous interventricular septum. A long-axis section through the interventricular septum in a heart with an aneurysm of the membranous septum. The original defect can be seen just below the aortic valve. It has been spontaneously closed by tricuspid valve tissue which still bulges into the right ventricular outflow forming the floor of an aneurysmal sac.

10.16 Self-closing ventricular septal defect. A ventricular septal defect viewed from the right side. The defect has been largely closed by adherence of the septal cusp of the tricuspid valve to its rim, leaving only a pin-point residual hole. This mechanism accounts for the spontaneous closure of a significant number of small holes in the first years of life. Growth and apposition of the muscular rim is another potential mechanism.

10.17 Surgical closure of ventricular septal defect. In closing ventricular septal defects the patch is sewn over the hole on the right side. Sutures are placed low in the septum to avoid the crest of the muscular septum. This crest contains the main atrioventricular bundle and is the inferior rim of the defect. Since the defect is closed from the right, as viewed from the left, a blind pocket is left whose floor is the patch. In this specimen, cut in a long axis view, such an aneurysm is present just below the aortic valve. It corresponds exactly to the aneurysm of the membranous septum following spontaneous closure.

10.18 Pulmonary vascular changes in ventricular septal defect. Muscular pulmonary artery in a patient with a large ventricular septal defect. There is very gross hypertrophy of medial smooth muscle which, in association with intimal thickening, has produced a very thick-walled vessel with a small lumen.
x175 Hematoxylin and eosin.

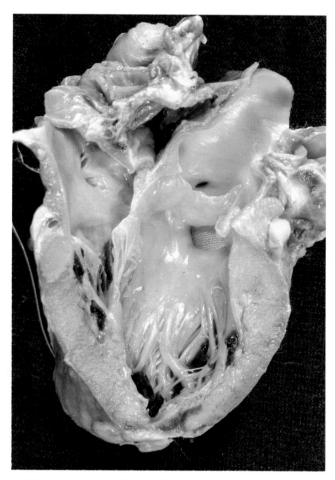

10.17 Surgical closure of septal defect

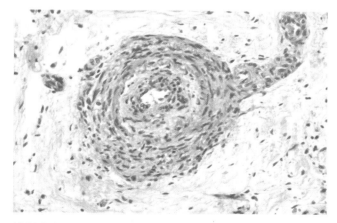

10.18 Pulmonary arteries: ventricular septal defect

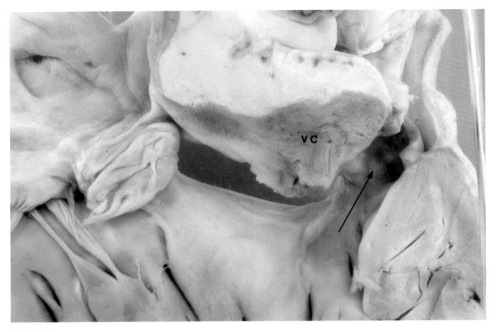

10.19 Fallot's tetralogy

10.19   Fallot's tetralogy. Fallot's tetralogy viewed from the right side. A large ventricular septal defect is visible beneath the supraventricular crest (VC). The right ventricular outflow (arrow) seen just anterior to the ridge is very narrow, due both to hypertrophy of the infundibular muscle and to valve stenosis with a very small main pulmonary artery. The two main components of the Fallot heart are thus present.

10.20   Fallot's tetralogy. Fallot's tetralogy viewed from the left side. There is a large aorta, and beneath the aortic valve is a large ventricular septal defect. The septal defect in this case comes up to the aortic valve with no intervening tissue. There is, therefore, a risk of aortic regurgitation. The aorta is large and appears shifted over to the right side of the interventricular septum. The aorta is not in line with the ventricular septum.

10.21   Fallot's tetralogy. The right ventricular outflow has been opened in a case of Fallot's tetralogy. The infundibular zone below the valve shows dense endocardial thickening, and the valve (PV) was a fibrous dome with a central hole. The combination of infundibular and valve stenosis is common in Fallot's tetralogy and, in addition, there may be hypoplasia of the main pulmonary trunk.

10.22   Repair of right ventricular outflow in Fallot's tetralogy. In extreme cases of Fallot's tetralogy the infundibular stenosis cannot be relieved by simply 'gouging' out muscle, since the whole outflow tract is hypoplastic. In these cases the outflow has to be enlarged by inserting a patch of pericardium.

10.23   Fallot's tetralogy. In this case there was stenosis purely at valve level. The pulmonary valve is viewed from above. The valve cusps are fused together to form a fibrous dome. At one edge there is a small eccentrically placed orifice.

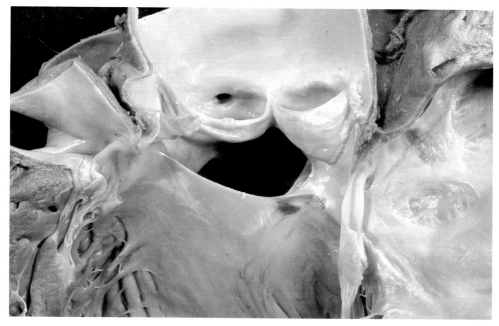

10.20 Fallot's tetralogy

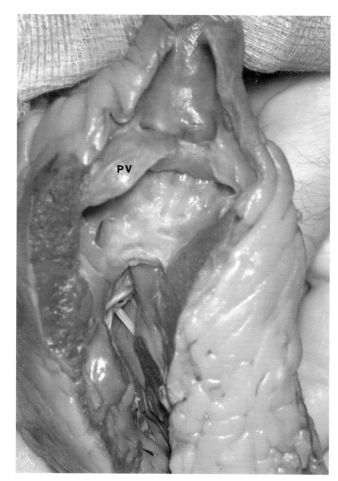

10.21 Fallot's tetralogy

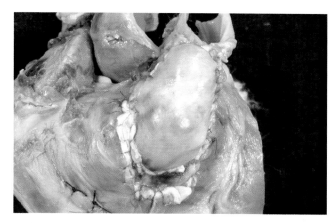

10.22 Right ventricular repair: Fallot's tetralogy

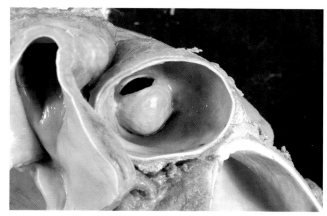

10.23 Fallot's tetralogy

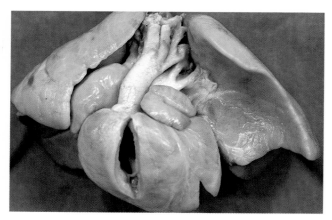

10.24 Complete transposition

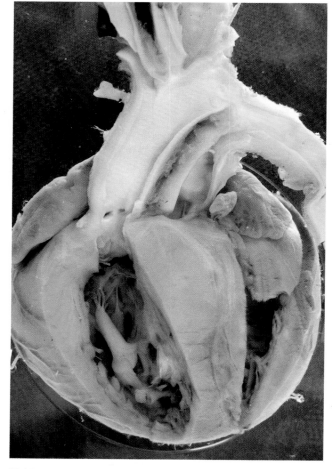

10.24 Complete transposition of the great vessels.
The specimen is viewed from the front and it can be seen that the aortic arch, identified by the carotid arteries, originates from the right ventricle.

10.25 Complete transposition of the great vessels.
The heart is viewed from the front with the main trunks opened. The trunk originating from the right ventricle has the coronary ostia and the vessels to the head and neck.

10.25 Complete transposition

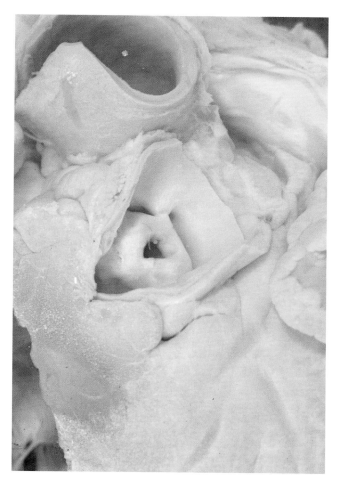

10.26 Isolated pulmonary stenosis

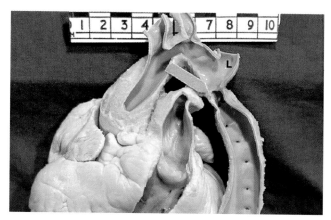

10.27 Coarctation

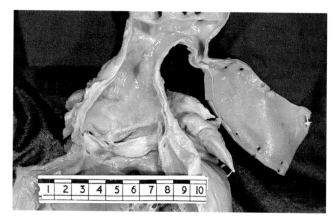

10.28 Coarctation

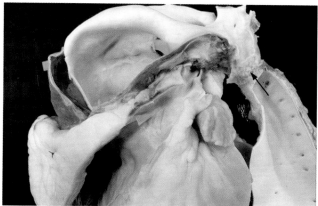

10.29 Coarctation

10.26   Isolated congenital pulmonary valve stenosis.
The pulmonary valve, which is viewed from above, is a
dome-shaped mass of fibrous tissue with a central opening
and small ridges marking where commissures should have
developed.

10.27   Coarctation of the aorta. There is a very distinct
localized stenosis of the aorta (red marker) just distal to
the left subclavian artery (L). The orifices of the intercostal
arteries in the descending aorta distal to the coarctation
are large due to the development of collateral blood flow.

10.28   Coarctation of the aorta. A coarctation of the
aorta which is just distal to the left subclavian artery (red
marker). The stenosis is very severe, reducing the lumen
to a tiny fissure. The ascending aorta is markedly dilated
and the aortic valve is bicuspid. Aortic regurgitation was
present in life. It is this type of case which runs a risk of
rupture of the ascending aorta.

10.29   Coarctation of the aorta. The aorta proximal to
the coarctation (arrow) is dilated and has a dissecting
aneurysm (orange marker) which had ruptured into the
pericardium and caused death. The intercostal artery
orifices are prominent.

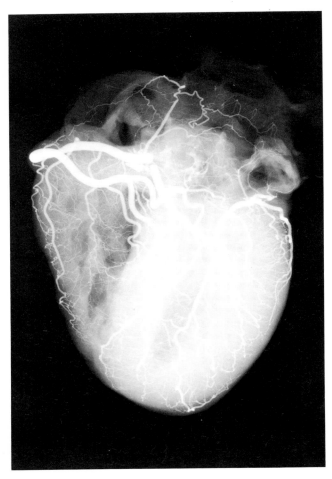

10.30 Single coronary artery

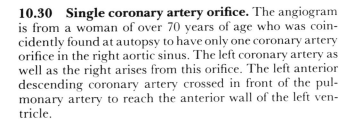

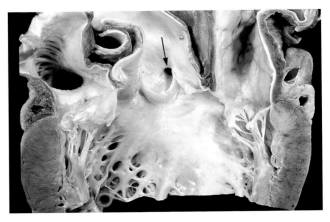

10.31 Anomalous coronary artery

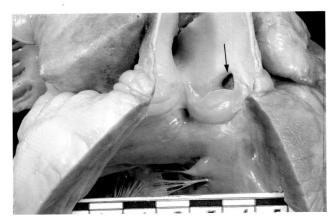

10.32 Anomalous coronary artery

10.30 Single coronary artery orifice. The angiogram is from a woman of over 70 years of age who was coincidently found at autopsy to have only one coronary artery orifice in the right aortic sinus. The left coronary artery as well as the right arises from this orifice. The left anterior descending coronary artery crossed in front of the pulmonary artery to reach the anterior wall of the left ventricle.

10.31 Anomalous origin of coronary artery. The patient died suddenly while training for a marathon race having been apparently fit. There is a single coronary artery orifice (arrow) in the aorta. The endocardium of the left ventricle over the septum is white and opaque.

10.32 Anomalous origin of coronary artery. The pulmonary artery has been opened anteriorly in the same case as **10.31**. The right coronary orifice (arrow) opens from the pulmonary artery.

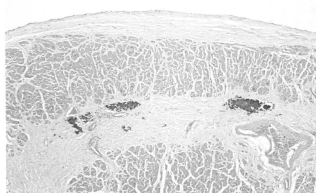

10.33 Myocardium: anomalous coronary artery

10.33 The myocardium in anomalous origin of the coronary artery. From the same case as **10.31** and **10.32**. There is a marked increase in fibrosis with focal areas of calcification in the subendocardial zone of the left ventricle. x18 Hematoxylin and eosin.

CHAPTER 11

Cardiac Surgery

VALVE SURGERY
(11.1 – 11.17)

Modern cardiac surgery has become so successful and widespread that some knowledge of its pathological sequelae is necessary.

Valve surgery initially consisted of relieving obstruction as rapidly as possible by valvotomy. To relieve congenital pulmonary valve stenosis the valve tissue was simply divided; the resultant pulmonary incompetence was trivial and inconsequential in patients without pulmonary hypertension. The operation was, and still is, highly successful. Aortic valvotomy, whether for congenital stenosis or for calcific aortic valve stenosis in adults, was not successful, largely because in the high pressure systemic circulation to leave a competent valve was essential and could not be achieved. Mitral valvotomy for rheumatic stenosis was highly successful when applied to valves which were not heavily calcified. It consisted of reopening the fused commissures with finger or dilator. When the valve was calcified or very densely fibrotic, considerable regurgitation was at times created and the results were less successful. Some control of incompetent mitral or tricuspid regurgitation valves due to ring dilatation, can be achieved by reducing the size of the valve orifice. But, in general, repair of incompetent valves has proved difficult.

The consequence of the failure of conservative valve surgery was the need to replace the whole valve with some form of prosthesis. Many prosthetic valves are in use, both mechanical and tissue. The aortic human homograft was a cadaver valve taken within 48 hours of death of the donor, kept in an antibiotic/nutrient medium and then inserted into the recipient, usually without use of a rigid frame. The end result, even after years, may closely resemble a normal valve. Other forms of tissue valve were constructed from pericardium or fascia from the patient, and used a rigid frame or stent. Heterograft valves are pig aortic cusps sewn within a rigid frame. The cusps are fixed in glutaraldehyde and are thus inert, making the term heterograft a misnomer. Such frame-supported valves can be used in either the mitral or the aortic position.

Mechanical valves come in many types. The most commonly used are the ball and cage variety and spring-loaded or sliding discs. In all of these there is a fabric covered valve ring sewn into the original valve ring after removing the abnormal cusps. The prosthetic valve ring rapidly becomes covered in a white fibrous new 'endothelium'.

The major complication of all tissue valves, whether homograft or heterograft, is progressive calcification of the cusps leading to stiffness and, finally, to cusp-tearing or even to complete cusp disintegration. The factors which encourage this process are presumably related to the handling and the nature of the donor tissue and to individual variations within the recipient. Any form of tissue valve which has been fixed in glutaraldehyde is dead, inert fibrous tissue. Claims have been made that in some instances fresh human homograft valves are viable and self replicate in the recipient, thus being true homografts. The consensus view is that these valves do not contain viable cells, and again the term homograft is inaccurate. An individual tendency for inert fibrous tissue to calcify is the major cause of graft failure and is very poorly understood.

Bacterial endocarditis is also a well-established risk of all tissue valves, but without infection thrombo-embolic complications are rare. In contrast, mechanical valves have a considerable and persistent risk of thrombo-embolism from small thrombi on the ring or cage. Infective endocarditis is also a continuing risk. Mechanical failure was formerly a risk, but has declined with better design of prosthesis and use of newer materials.

With either tissue or mechanical valves used in the mitral position, thrombosis may develop in the left atrium and lead to obstruction of the valve orifice. The sutures used around the prosthetic valve ring may dehisce from the native ring into which they are inserted. Massive displacement can occur, with tilting of the whole prosthesis. If only one or two sutures are torn out, a chronic para-valve leak may be established. Through these defects high-pressure flow occurs, with destruction of red cells and a hemolytic anemia develops, with hemosiderin detectable in the urine and renal tubules.

SURGERY FOR ISCHEMIC HEART DISEASE
(11.18 – 11.28)

The earliest attempts at myocardial revascularization included induction of pericardial adhesions and the Weinberg procedure, in which the cut end of an internal mammary artery was simply buried in the myocardium. Minor myocardial vascularization was achieved, but the operation was not widely regarded as a success. Coronary artery by-pass grafting (CABG) has become the most widely practised cardiac operation. In this procedure lengths of the patient's own saphenous vein are reversed (because of venous valves) and anastomosed from the ascending aorta to the coronary arteries distal to an obstruction. Segments of the internal mammary artery have also been used by some surgeons. Multiple side-to-side anastomoses to the coronary arteries may be made from one proximal anastomosis. The operation has a low mortality; such perioperative deaths as do occur usually result from acute myocardial infarction developing at the time of graft insertion. The more proximal the stenotic lesions that are being by-passed, and the more free of atheroma the distal vessel, the greater is the chance of long-term graft function. Around 85% of grafts can be shown to be patent at 6 months. Acute occlusion of the graft at operation usually follows poor distal run-off, i.e. a very small distal lumen through which flow is small, dissection into the media at the distal anastomosis site, or following endarterectomy undertaken when the lumen is too small for initial grafting.

In the first 3 months the vein undergoes a series of adaptive changes to high pressure flow. These consist of intimal smooth muscle and elastic deposition in which the incorporation of small platelet thrombi seems important. Clinical studies suggest that the use of antiplatelet drugs enhances graft patency.

Occlusion of a graft which has functioned for some months may be associated with low flow due to progressive atheromatous disease in the distal part of the native grafted vessel or with development of atheroma in the graft itself. This is a very diffuse insudation of lipid into the superficial layers of the intima. True plaque formation is rare. The lipid-containing layer of the intima breaks up, leading to occlusion of the lumen by a complex mixture of lipid and thrombus.

11.1   Post commissurotomy mitral valve. Mitral valve viewed from the left atrium from a patient who had a closed valvotomy for mitral stenosis some years previously. There are sharp-edged, V-shaped cuts still visible in the commissural areas. Restenosis has not occurred in this case but is a well-recognized risk.

11.2   Aortic valve homograft. Aortic homograft valve after being in situ and functioning normally for some years. The valve has been opened to show that the cusps are intact and pliable. Apart from the intimal thickening over the upper suture line, which can just be seen, the valve looks very like a normal valve. A coronary vein graft orifice (arrow) is also present just alongside the aortotomy recognized by the suture material beneath the intima.

11.3   Heterograft prosthetic valve. A Carpentier-Edwards heterograft valve which is derived from a pig aortic valve and contained within a rigid stent which has a cloth covered ring. The valve is viewed from the proximal side as regards blood flow. The valve can be used in the mitral or aortic position.

11.4   Heterograft valve in the mitral position. A Carpentier-Edwards heterograft inserted into the mitral position viewed from the opposite i.e. distal face from **11.3**. The stent has three sharp points to which the cusp commissures are attached.

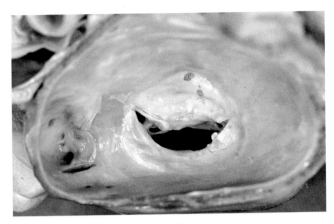

11.1 Post commissurotomy mitral valve

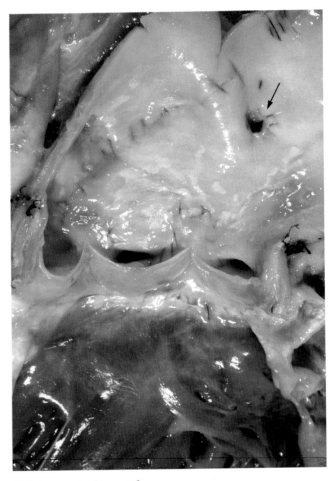

11.2 Aortic valve homograft

11.5   Ball and cage prosthetic valve. A Starr-Edwards prosthetic valve in the mitral position viewed from the left ventricle. The ball is silastic in this case although metal balls are also used. The cage projects into the cavity of the left ventricle. Considerable white endocardial thickening has occurred over the cut stumps of the papillary muscles.

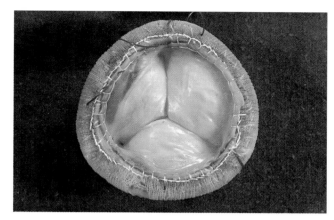

11.3 Heterograft prosthetic valve

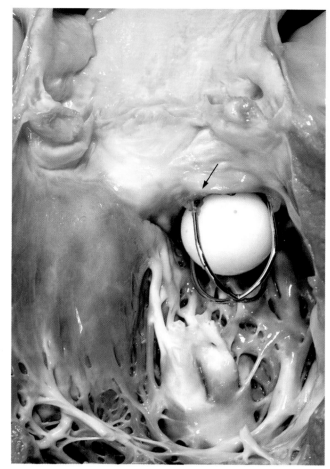

11.5 Ball and cage valve

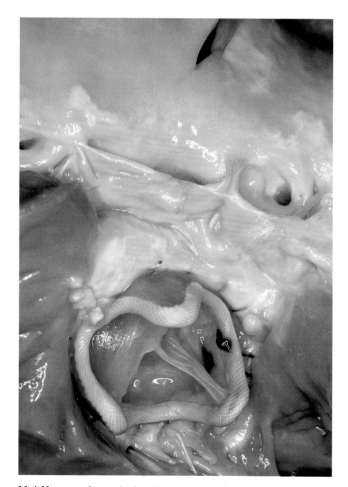

11.4 Heterograft prosthetic valve

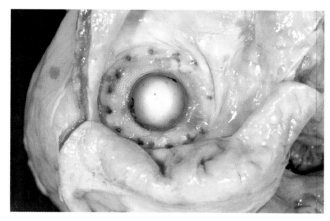

11.6 Ball and cage valve

Small fragments of thrombus (arrow) are present on the cage. The aortic valve has not been replaced but does show some cusp fibrosis due to chronic rheumatic disease.

11.6 Ball and cage prosthetic valve. A Starr-Edwards prosthetic valve in the mitral position viewed from the left atrium. The valve has been in situ some months and the ring is partially covered by a 'new' endocardium. The sutures still remain visible sticking through the endothelium and do so for years. In some areas the teflon of the sewing ring has not become covered by endothelium.

11.7 Disc type prosthesis. A tilting spring-loaded disc-type prosthetic valve in the mitral position. The advantage of this valve is that it is flat without a cage impinging on the left ventricle as it contracts.

11.8 Heterograft prosthetic failure. Five years after insertion, this pig heterograft valve developed severe calcification leading to severe mitral stenosis.

11.9 Heterograft prosthetic valve failure. Heterograft pig valve excised following mitral regurgitation which developed three years after insertion. The cusps were yellow and evenly calcified with tearing of two cusps. This cusp calcification is the long term complication responsible for most failure of this type of valve. Children appear to develop cusp calcification more rapidly than adults.

11.10 Ball cage valve obstruction. Starr-type cage and ball valve in the mitral position viewed from the left atrium. A fringe of thrombus has developed on the ring projecting across into the valve orifice. This leads to obstruction and a clinical picture akin to mitral stenosis.

11.11 Disc-type prosthetic valve failure. Disc-type prosthesis in which constant movement has eroded a V-shaped groove into the edge of the disc. Mechanical failure of prosthetic valves include the disc or the ball jamming, leading to acute obstruction or to actual disintegration of the ball with severe regurgitation. In the period before the balls were metal, insudation of lipid led to ball swelling and jamming in the cage.

11.12 and 11.13 Prosthetic valve obstruction. Massive atrial thrombosis (**11.12**) developing as a pannus over the orifice of a pig heterograft valve three days after successful mitral valve replacement. The thrombus could be flapped over easily to display the valve (**11.13**). In life, obstruction was intermittent. Such massive thrombosis often follows low cardiac output in the post-operative phase.

11.14 Prosthetic valve dehiscence. Acute dehiscence of a heterograft valve over one edge (arrows) due to the ring sutures cutting through, leading to severe regurgitation soon after operation.

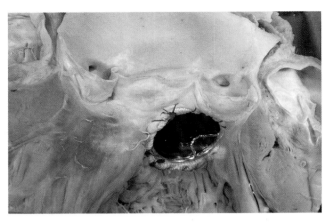

11.7 Disc type prosthesis

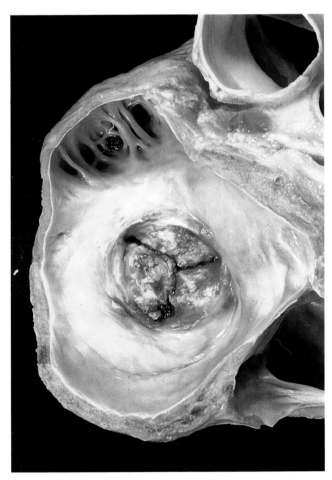

11.8 Heterograft valve failure

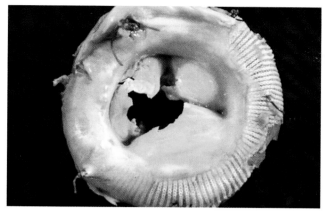

11.9 Heterograft valve failure

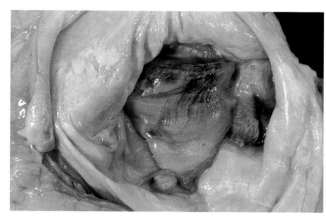

11.12 Prosthetic valve obstruction

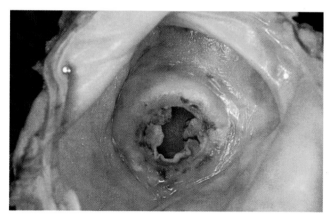

11.10 Ball valve obstruction

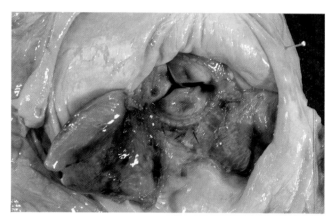

11.13 Prosthetic valve obstruction

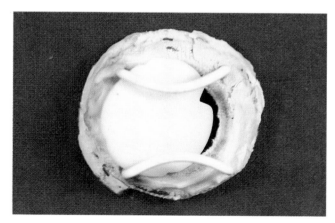

11.11 Disc-type valve failure

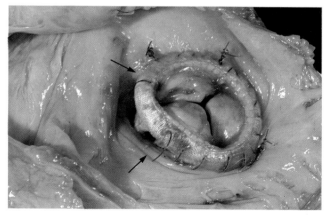

11.14 Prosthetic valve dehiscence

11.15 Prosthetic para-valve leakage. Chronic para-valve leak in a Starr-type prosthesis in the mitral position. One suture had cut through, leading to a small hole (red marker) alongside the valve ring. Very high pressure regurgitant jets develop through such holes. The remainder of the ring is covered with endothelium and free of thrombus.

11.16 Hemolytic anemia in para-valve leakage. The kidney from the patient whose valve is shown in **11.15**. The renal tubules stain an intense blue due to iron deposition. Hemolytic anemia present in life. The hemolytic anemia results from mechanical trauma to red blood cells in the high-pressure regurgitant jet.
x95 Perls' stain

11.17 Post cardiac surgery diffuse myocardial necrosis. Hemorrhagic necrosis throughout the whole subendocardial zone in a patient who failed to survive cardio-pulmonary by-pass due to myocardial damage. This pattern of necrosis develops particularly in association with severe left ventricular hypertrophy as, for example, aortic valve stenosis, but it also complicates vein graft operations. It is an overall failure of myocardial perfusion not relating to only one graft.

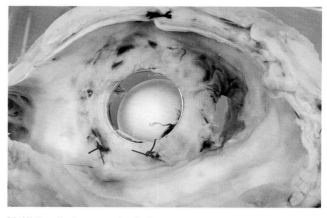

11.15 Prosthetic para-valve leakage

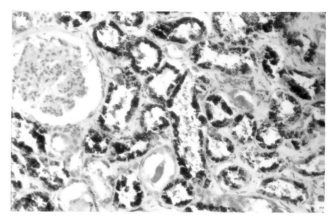

11.16 Hemolytic anemia: para-valve leakage

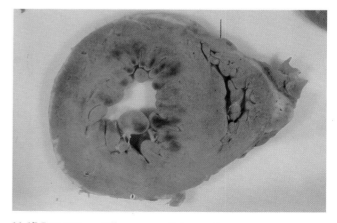

11.17 Post surgery diffuse myocardial necrosis

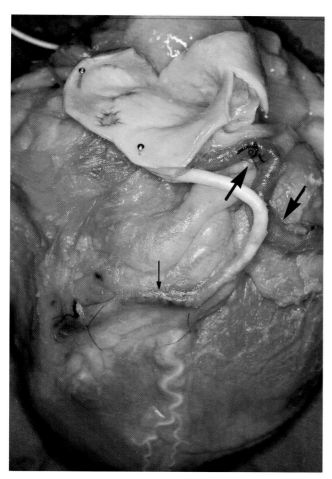

11.18 Coronary vein grafts

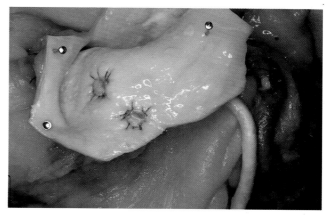

11.19 Coronary vein grafts

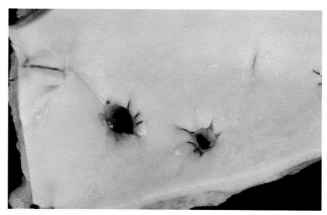

11.20 Coronary vein grafts

11.18   Coronary vein grafts. Coronary vein grafts in a patient who died soon after surgery. There is one patent graft which contains barium injection media. This graft can be seen to fill one coronary artery by a side-to-side anastomosis. The continuation of the graft to another coronary vessel (thin arrow), however, contains thrombus and has not filled. A second graft from the aorta (thick arrows) is distended by recent thrombus. Acute thrombosis of grafts immediately after operation is associated with poor distal flow ('run-off') usually due to grafting severely narrowed arteries.

11.19   Coronary vein grafts. The aortic openings of two vein grafts at one day after insertion. The suture lines are clearly seen.

11.20   Coronary vein grafts. The aortic openings of two vein grafts three years after insertion. The orifices are widely patent and the suture lines partially covered by a new intimal layer. However, the sutures are still clearly recognizable.

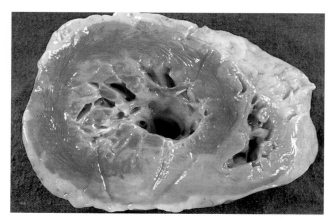

11.21 Post operative myocardial infarction

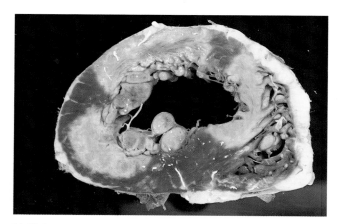

11.22 Post operative myocardial infarction

11.21   Post operative myocardial infarction in vein grafts. Hemorrhagic infarction following graft insertion for acute coronary thrombosis. The hemorrhage results from reperfusing ischemically-damaged vessels in the necrotic area of myocardium. A similar form of myocardial infarction characterized by intense intra-myocardial bleeding results from thrombolysis of acute thrombi which has caused infarction.

11.22   Post operative myocardial infarction. Three separate regional infarcts developing after insertion of triple vein grafts. Transverse slice of myocardium stained for succinic dehydrogenase activity. The areas of infarction are pale as compared to the dark blue stained normal myocardium. These discrete regional areas of necrosis suggest technical difficulty or perioperative thrombosis in the graft supplying these areas. The commonest cause of perioperative death in vein graft operations is myocardial infarction.

11.23   Vein graft anastomosis. Transverse histological section across an anastomosis of vein graft to coronary artery in a patient who died within days. The anastomosis is widely patent. The vein (V) has a thin fibrous wall; the artery (A) is also normal. Both have been opened and sutured together. The suture material can be seen (arrows).

11.24   Vein graft anastomosis. Section across an anastomosis associated with low flow in the post operative phase. The vein graft (V) is thin-walled and patent, but the arterial wall (A) has gross intimal thickening due to atheroma at the anastomosis site. The picture illustrates the technical difficulty in grafting into severely diseased arteries.

11.25   Vein graft anastomosis three years after insertion. Section across a functional anastomosis three years after insertion. The sutures (arrows) mark the junction between artery and vein. The vein wall (V) is thickened as compared to **11.23** and **11.24** due to a new intimal layer of smooth muscle. The residual portion of arterial wall (A) shows an atheromatous plaque.

11.26, 11.27   Long term functional vein graft. The wall of a functional vein graft at three years. The media (M) of the vein contains irregular elastic laminae. The thickening of the wall is seen to be internal to this zone and is composed predominantly of smooth muscle several times thicker than the media. (Lumen – L).
11.26 x95 Hematoxylin and eosin.
11.27 x95 Elastic-van Gieson.

11.28   Vein graft atheroma. Vein graft atheroma developing after four years of function. The graft wall is thickened. The intima is now predominantly comprised of collagen. In the superficial layer of the intima, lipid is contained within foamy histiocytic cells. Massive thrombosis follows break up of the superficial layers exposing the lipid to the blood flow.
x60 Hematoxylin and eosin.

References:

Ionescu M I ed. Tissue Heart Valves. London: Butterworths 1979.

Longmore D B ed. Modern Cardiac Surgery. England: MTP Press 1978.

Silver M D ed. in Cardiovascular Pathology. New York: Churchill Livingstone 1983.

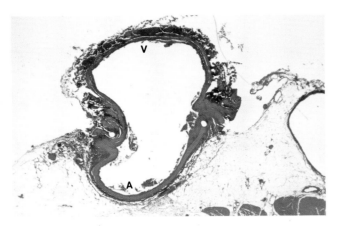

11.23 Vein graft anastomosis

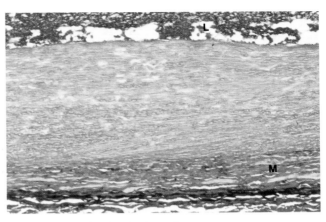

11.26 Long term functional vein graft

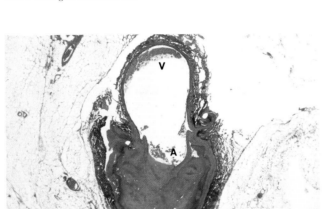

11.24 Vein graft anastomosis

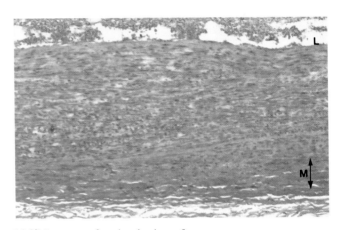

11.27 Long term functional vein graft

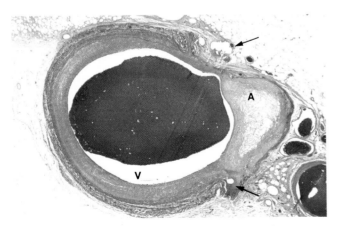

11.25 Vein graft anastomosis

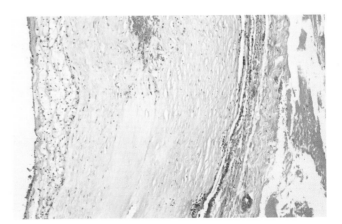

11.28 Vein graft atheroma

APPENDIX 1

Examination of the Conduction System

Successful examination requires considerable knowledge of cardiac anatomy to ensure that the blocks are correctly taken and orientated, as well as the ability to recognize conduction fibres histologically. It is not an easy task, and the best advice to anyone wishing to examine pathological material is to first study a large number of normal hearts. There are considerable age-related changes in the conduction system, and knowledge of these is essential to avoid over-interpretation of morphological changes. The morphological responses of conduction fibres are limited and can be succinctly expressed as being either present or absent. In the latter case, certainty of their absence entails tracing the conduction system from where it is normal into the area of destruction; thus some form of step or serial sectioning is mandatory. Some indication of the blocks taken to illustrate the conduction system will be given, along with a brief account of the normal appearances. The

reader is referred to detailed texts on the conduction system for further help. It should also be stated that studying conduction systems where no electrocardiographic data is available is of very limited use.

SINUS NODE (A1.1 – A1.4)

The sinus node lies in the junction of the superior vena cava and right atrium (A1.1). The nodal artery circles this junction and the node is arranged around it, close to where the crest of the atrial appendage joins the caval ring.

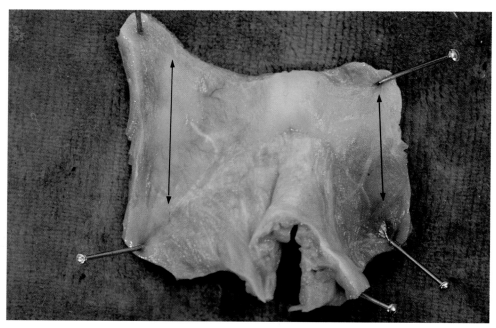

A1.1 Histological examination: sinus node

A1.1 Histological examination of sinus node. For histological study, the sino-caval ring is removed with an inch of tissue on either side. The ring is opened posteriorly and the tissue pinned flat. After fixation, blocks are taken in the longitudinal plane (arrow); those blocks around and lateral to the crest of the atrial appendage will contain the node. It cannot be identified by the naked eye. The nodal artery, particularly if distended by barium, can be easily seen and does indicate the site of the node.

A1.2 Histological appearance of normal sinus node. The nodal artery can be recognized by containing injection media (arrow). Around the artery is a mass of connective tissue within which are embedded numerous interweaving small cardiac muscle fibres. At the edge of the node there are numerous nerve bundles (N).
x125 Hematoxylin and eosin.

A1.3 Normal sinus node. In this trichrome-stained histological section of a normal sinus node, the muscle fibres can be more easily appreciated staining red in contrast to the blue staining collagenous stroma. This amount of fibrous stroma is normal within nodal tissue.
x125 Picro-Mallory trichrome.

A1.4 Sinus node in long-standing atrial fibrillation. In this trichrome-stained section the nodal artery can be recognized to be surrounded by a collagenous stroma, but fewer muscle fibres can be seen. This loss of specialized conduction fibres within the node is associated with all forms of sinoatrial disease. It is virtually the only morphological response that nodal tissue undergoes, apart from replacement by amyloid. With increasing age, even in asymptomatic normal individuals, the proportion of nodal muscle within the node falls, probably accounting for the frequency that atrial arrhythmias develop in old age.
x125 Picro-Mallory trichrome.

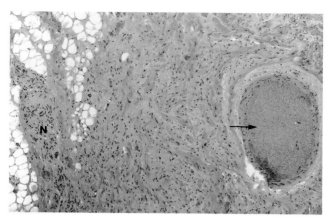

A1.2 Normal sinus node

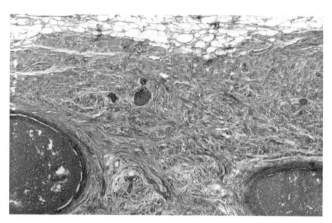

A1.3 Normal sinus node

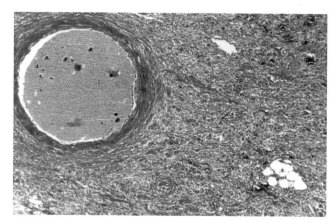

A1.4 Sinus node: atrial fibrillation

ATRIOVENTRICULAR
CONDUCTION SYSTEM
(A1.5 – A1.15)

To study the atrioventricular conduction system the lateral walls of the atria and ventricles are removed, isolating the interatrial and interventricular septae which are then fixed flat. It is difficult to achieve a good study of the conduction system in a heart which has been fixed by immersion of the whole specimen. Viewing the specimen from the right side, a central block of tissue is isolated which contains the A-V node, atrioventricular bundle and the proximal bundle branches. This central block is subdivided into smaller blocks which are step or serially sectioned from the posterior face. The conduction system is easily identified in ordinary hematoxylin and eosin-stained sections, but any of the trichrome stains differentiating muscle from collagen can be helpful.

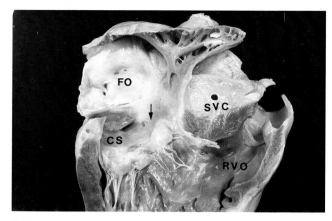

A1.5 Histological study: conduction system

A1.5 Tissue block taken to study the conduction system. The interatrial and interventricular septae are viewed from the right side. The atrioventricular node (arrow) is just anterior to the coronary sinus beneath the right atrial endocardium. (FO=foramen ovale, CS=coronary sinus, SVC=supra ventricular crest, RVO=right ventricular outflow).

A1.6 Tissue blocks taken to study the conduction system. From the large block of tissue shown in **A1.5**, a smaller oblong block is prepared. To do this, the tissue posterior to the coronary sinus, above the foramen ovale anterior to the supraventricular crest and below the mid point of the ventricular septum is removed. This is best achieved with a long (20cm) sharp knife. The block of tissue produced contains the membranous septum crossed by the septal cusp of the tricuspid valve (TV). This block is sectioned in the long axis beginning at the posterior border (arrow). Successive sections will pass through the node, main bundle and bundle branches. The block is too large for anything other than hand processing, and can be divided into up to 8 blocks. Trimming of each block will inevitably lose some tissue, so the number should be kept to a minimum. One transverse block across the lower portion of the ventricular septum is taken from the block to demonstrate the left bundle branch in cross section.

A1.7 Tissue blocks taken to study the conduction system. The same block as shown in **A1.6** is viewed from the left. The correct block will contain the aortic valve (A) with its continuity with the anterior cusp of the mitral valve (M). The membranous septum is in the angle between the aortic valve and the base of the anterior cusp of the mitral valve. The atrioventricular bundle of His runs on the crest of the muscular interventricular septum (arrow) inferior to the edge of the membranous septum.

A1.8 Normal atrioventricular node. The node (N) lies immediately beneath the right atrial endocardium adjacent to the central fibrous body (CFB) of the heart. It is a mass of interweaving small muscle fibres in structure akin to the sinus node but the connective tissue stroma is less dense. The central artery is a less constant feature in the atrioventricular node and often penetrates the central fibrous body to enter the upper ventricular septum leaving the node.
x100 Picro-Mallory trichrome.

A1.9 Normal atrioventricular bundle. The conduction system at this level consists of a single strand of muscle (arrows) embedded within the central fibrous body itself; hence it is often called the penetrating bundle. The atrioventricular bundle forms the only electrical connection between the atria and ventricle in normal hearts.
x25 Picro-Mallory trichrome.

A1.10 Normal bifurcating atrioventricular bundle. The main atrioventricular bundle lies at the crest of the muscular interventricular septum (IVS). The membranous septum (MS) a simple sheet of fibrous tissue lies above. The main bundle has given origin to the first of the slender left bundle branches which runs down the muscular septum immediately beneath the endocardium on the left side (arrows).
x35 Picro-Mallory trichrome.

References:

Davies M J, Anderson R H and Becker A E. The Conduction System of the Heart. London: Butterworths 1983.

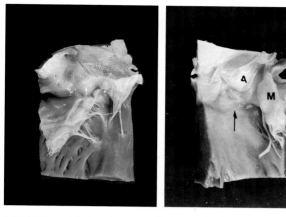

A1.6,7 Tissue blocks taken to study the conduction system

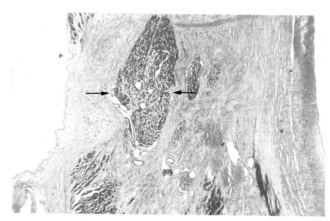

A1.9 Normal atrioventricular bundle

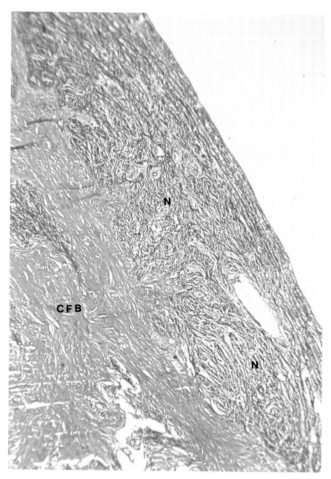

A1.8 Normal atrioventricular node

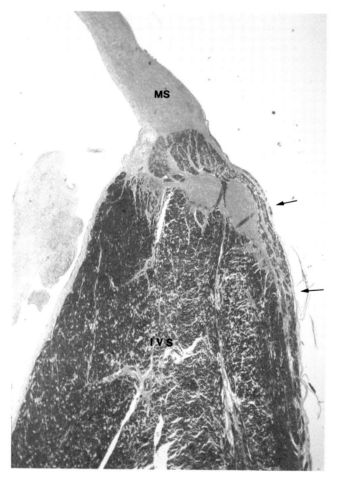

A1.10 Normal bifurcating atrioventricular bundle

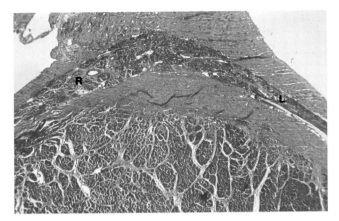

A1.11 Normal bifurcating bundle

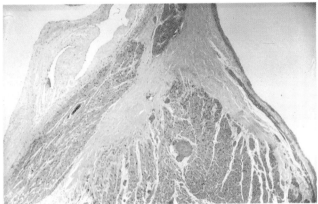

A1.12 Normal bundle branches

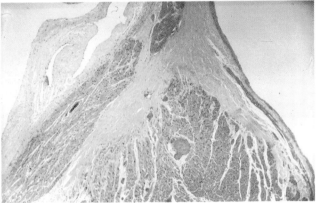

A1.13 Idiopathic bundle branch fibrosis

A1.11   Normal bifurcating atrioventricular bundle.
At this level the bundle still lies on the crest of the muscular
interventricular septum, and is beginning to bifurcate into
left and right bundle branches. The right (R) is a single
muscle bundle, the left branch (L) is made up of numerous
finer branches, only one of which is seen in this level.
x25 Picro-Mallory trichrome.

A1.12   Normal bundle branches. At this level the right
branch is now a separate mass of muscle passing down the
right side of the septum. A left fascicle is also present. In
all the sections **A1.9-A1.12** the conduction system is
encased in fibrous tissue which insulates it from the contractile myocardium.
x25 Picro-Mallory trichrome.

A1.13   Idiopathic bundle branch fibrosis. The right
branch (arrows) can be recognized by its outline and
position just beneath the endocardium on the right side of
the muscular interventricular septum. It contains a
reduced population of conduction fibres but no inflammatory cells. This condition, in which specialized conduction fibres simply vanish over some years, is a common
cause of complete heart block and is of unknown etiology.
x60 Hematoxylin and eosin.

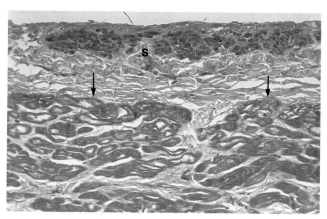

A1.15 Peripheral conduction fibres: man

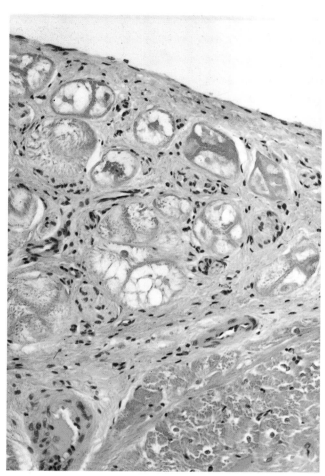

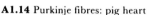

A1.14 Purkinje fibres: pig heart

A1.14   Purkinje fibres in the pig heart. In mammalian hearts the bundle branches end in a complex ramification of specialized muscle fibres which lie just beneath the endocardium and spread over the whole inner surface of both ventricles. In large mammals these cells have a very striking appearance, forming a subendocardial layer of very large, vacuolated cells which contain very few myofibrils. The myogenic nature of these cells is not easily apparent and was not realized by Purkinje, who described them in the pig in the nineteenth century.
x425 Hematoxylin and eosin.

A1.15   Peripheral conduction fibres in man. In man, the distal conduction fibres form a layer (arrows) just beneath the endocardium. They are somewhat larger and more vacuolated than contraction fibres, but the difference is not great. It is debated whether they should be called Purkinje fibres or not. They have the same function as the cells described by Purkinje but not the same morphology. Immediately beneath the endothelium of the endocardium is a layer of smooth muscle (S). This must not be mistaken for the layer of much larger conduction fibres.
x95 Picro-Mallory trichrome.

APPENDIX 2

Demonstration of Myocardial Infarction

The aim of techniques for demonstration of infarction is twofold; first, to identify necrosis at a stage at which it cannot be discerned by naked eye or microscopic examination and, second, to delineate exactly the areas of necrosis. The first is difficult, the second readily achieved.

Using slices of fresh myocardium, 1cm thick, usually taken through the short axis of the ventricles, there are a number of enzyme techniques described which will macroscopically identify normal muscle by the development of a colour reaction, and areas of infarction in which colour does not develop. All these techniques use a substrate which is broken down by dehydrogenases or other enzymes present in the normal myocardium, liberating H ions which then generate a colour reaction. The succinic dehydrogenase method using nitro blue tetrazolium (NBT) was adopted in this atlas (6.35-6.40, 6.62), but all the techniques are equally valid. The end point can be judged in two ways, either as areas of myocardium which develops a colour more slowly, or as areas which do not develop any colour. The former does have a subjective bias, but can detect early infarction; the latter is a reproducible method of delineating areas of infarction over 8-12 hours in age.

Microscopic methods of identifying early necrosis are widely described; but all suffer from a subjective element in that negative or positive results can be obtained at the wish of the technician carrying out the staining. Knowledge of what answer is required is a prerequisite of successful use of these techniques. They can all be made so sensitive that agonal changes in the myocardium are demonstrated.

The methods largely depend on the altered affinity of the myofibrils in ischemic muscle cells to take up eosin or basic fuchsin dye (6.44). The method used personally is shown below, but there is no inherent reason to suppose any method is superior to another.

Other techniques in addition to these staining methods include biochemical estimation of the Na^+ to K^+ ratio of different zones of the myocardium, and the detection of alterations in the autofluorescence of hematoxylin and eosin stained sections and wavy fibres (6.44). All are regarded as useful and specific by their protagonists but, again, will detect agonal and autolytic changes making their specificity less than absolute.

References:

Anderson K R, Popple A, Parker D J, Sayer R, Trickey R J and Davies M J. An experimental assessment of the macroscopic enzyme techniques for the autopsy demonstration of myocardial infarction. J Pathol 1979; 127: 93-98.

Lie J T, Holley K, Kampa W R and Titus J L. New histochemical method for morphological diagnosis of early stages of myocardial ischaemia. Mayo Clinic Proceedings 1971; 46: 319-327.

DEMONSTRATION OF SUCCINIC DEHYDROGENASE IN TISSUE SLICES

Stock solution A: Nitro-blue tetrazolium 1mg/ml in distilled water.

Stock solution B: Phosphate buffered saline (pH 7.3). Use Oxoid Dulbecco A tablets. For use, add 30ml of solution A to 70ml of solution B, and add a pinch of sodium succinate. After mixing, immerse the tissue slice in this solution and watch for colour development. The reaction is stopped by immersing the slice in formal saline. Care must be taken that the solution completely covers the tissue. The reaction is accelerated by temperature, but at room temperature a colour will develop in 10-15 minutes. Colour will develop, but more slowly, if the succinate is omitted from the incubation medium. The method is relatively unaffected by autolysis, but the first indication that this is present is a reduction in staining over the right ventricle.

BASIC FUCHSIN STAIN FOR EARLY INFARCTION

Staining solutions:

Solution A: Alum hematoxylin. Mix 6g of aluminium sulphate, 0.5g of hematoxylin and 0.25g of yellow mercuric oxide in 70ml of distilled water. Boil for 10 minutes. Cool and then add 30ml of glycerine and 4ml of glacial acetic acid. Filter before use.

Solution B. 0.1% basic fuchsin in distilled water.

Solution C. 0.1% picric acid in absolute acetone.

Staining procedure

Deparaffinize section and hydrate to distilled water. Stain in solution A for 10 seconds. Wash in running cold tap water for 5 minutes. Stain in solution B for 3 minutes. Rinse for 5-10 seconds in distilled water and again in absolute acetone. Differentiate in solution C until the red (basic fuchsin) colour ceases to run off the section - usually about 20 seconds. Rinse for 5-10 seconds in absolute acetone, clear in xylol and mount in a resinous mounting medium. Counterstain cytoplasm as preferred.

A 2.1 Appearances of tissue

Crimson red:- ischemic myocardial cells.

Light blue:- normal myocardial cells.

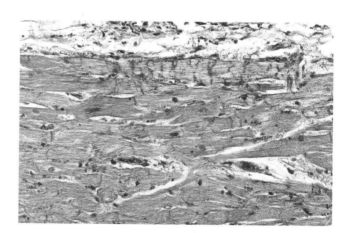

APPENDIX 3

Assessment of Cardiac Hypertrophy at Autopsy

The methods available are:

(1) Total heart weight

The total weight of the fresh or fixed heart is recorded after opening the chambers to remove blood clot. The advantage of this method is the ease with which the measurement is made, but the limitations of the data obtained must be, and rarely are, appreciated. There is a linear relation between isolated left ventricular mass and total heart weight, largely dependent on the fact that the former is the largest component of the latter. There is no relation of isolated right ventricular mass to total heart weight. In considering any individual total heart weight, allowance must be made for body size in deciding whether cardiomegaly is present. Total heart weight correlates most closely with total body weight rather than with height.

Thus the total heart weight can give a valuable indication of left ventricular hypertrophy, but can give no indication of right ventricular hypertrophy and *must* always be judged in relation to body weight.

In the following tables the mean and the 95% confidence upper limit of heart and ventricular weights is given for clinically normal individuals with regard to their body mass. In this and any other quoted range of heart weights, unrecognized hypertension may be responsible for the difficulty in defining in the upper limit of normality. When body weight is taken into account, atrophic hearts, i.e. those falling below the limit of normal heart weight are rare. It is true that trained athletes have increased heart weights, but otherwise physical activity seems of little relevance in determining heart weight.

(2) Isolated ventricular weights (7.3)

In the method described by Fulton both ventricles are dissected out independently, and the weight of each recorded. Epicardial fat is scraped away and the atria removed. The interventricular septum is taken as being a part of the left ventricle. The method can be performed easily only on formalin-fixed hearts, and takes approximately 10 minutes per specimen; its advantage is the ability to determine the mass of each ventricle independently, and it is virtually the only method of accurately measuring right ventricular hypertrophy.

The normal ranges must again be modified in respect of total body weight. In cases where both ventricles are increased in weight the ratio of right to left indicates which ventricle is most severely affected. The normal ratio is 2.5-3.5.

(3) Ventricular wall thickness

This method is widely used, quite unjustifiably; its sole merit being the ease with which the measurement is made. The measurements obtained are not reproducible between observers and correlate very poorly with ventricular mass. The major reason for this disappointing fact is that wall thickness depends on another variable, cavity size, for which measurement is very difficult. It cannot be sufficiently emphasized that many hearts apparently arrest in systole rigor. The LV wall thickness may be over 2cm with a small cavity and a normal LV mass. At the other extreme, in a dilated heart a left ventricle with an isolated mass over 300g may have a wall thickness of 1cm.

Predicted upper limit of heart weight, L.V. weight and R.V. weight with 95% C.I. for prediction

FEMALE			MALE		
Body weight (kg)	Mean (g)	95% C.I. Upper (g)	Body weight (kg)	Mean (g)	95% C.I. Upper (g)
Total heart weight			**Total heart weight**		
30	224	273	30		
40	268	302	40	287	342
50	313	339	50	320	360
60	357	391	60	354	382
70	401	450	70	387	403
80			80	420	454
90			90	454	502
L.V. weight			**L.V. weight**		
30	99	116	30		
40	112	124	40	124	140
50	125	135	50	140	151
60	138	149	60	157	165
70	151	166	70	173	182
80			80	190	203
90			90	207	225
R.V. weight			**R.V. weight**		
30	33	38	30		
40	36	40	40	37	45
50	39	42	50	43	49
60	43	47	60	49	53
70	46	51	70	54	58
80			80	60	65
90			90	66	71

Bibliography

Adler, C P, Morphometric and Cytophometric Investigations of Myocardial Diseases. In H Just, Schuster H P, eds., Myocarditis and Cardiomyopathy, Berlin: Springer 1983; 143-181.

Anderson R H and Becker A E. Cardiac Anatomy. London: Gower Medical Publishing; Edinburgh: Churchill Livingstone 1980.

Anderson R H, Becker A E, Lucchese F E, Meier M A, Rogby M L and Soto B. Morphology of Congenital Heart Disease. Tunbridge Wells: Castle House 1983.

Anderson K R, Popple A, Parker D J, Sayer R, Trickey R J and Davies M J. An experimental assessment of the macroscopic enzyme techniques for the autopsy demonstration of myocardial infarction. J Pathol 1979; 127: 93-98.

Ansell B M and Simkin P A eds. The Heart and Rheumatic Disease. London: Butterworths 1984.

Bayliss R, Clarke C, Oakley C M, Somerville W and Whitefield A G W. The teeth and infective endocarditis. Br Heart J 1983; 50: 506-512.

Bayliss R, Clarke C, Oakley C M, Somerville W, Whitefield A G W and Young S E J. The microbiology and pathogenesis of infective endocarditis. Br Heart J 1983; 50: 513-519.

Bayliss R, Clarke C, Oakley C M, Somerville W, Whitefield A G W and Young S E J. The bowel, the genitourinary tract, and infective endocarditis. Br Heart J 1984; 51: 339-345.

Becker A E and Anderson R H. Pathology of Congenital Heart Disease. London: Butterworths 1981.

Becker A E and Anderson R H. Cardiac Pathology. Edinburgh: Churchill Livingstone 1984.

Becker A E and Caruso G. Myocardial disarray. A critical review. Br Heart J 1982; 104: 155-155.

Becker A E. Myocarditis. In Silver M D ed. Cardiovascular Pathology. New York: Churchill Livingstone 1983; 469-489.

Billingham M E. Some recent advances in cardiac pathology. Human Pathology 1979; 10: 367-387.

Brigden W. Uncommon myocardial diseases. The non-coronary cardiomyopathies. Lancet 1957; 2: 1179-1184.

Bruton D, Herdson P B and Beecroft D M O. Histiocytoid cardiomyopathy of infancy: an unexplained myofibre degeneration. Pathology 1977; 9: 123-125.

Bulkley B H and Roberts W C. Ankylosing spondylitis and aortic regurgitation – description of the characteristic cardiovascular lesion from study of eight necropsy patients. Circulation 1973; 48: 1014-1027.

Bulkley B H and Roberts W C. The heart in systemic lupus erythematosus and the changes induced in it by cortico steroid therapy – a study of 36 necropsy patients. Am J Med 1975; 58: 243-264.

Bulkley B H and Roberts W C. Dilatation of the mitral annulus. A rare cause of mitral regurgitation. Am J Med 1975; 59: 457-463.

Burch G E, Depasquale N P and Phillips J H. The syndrome of papillary muscle dysfunction. Am Heart J 1968; 75: 399-415.

Burch G E and Giles T D. Angle of traction of the papillary muscles on normal and dilated hearts. A theoretical analysis of its importance in mitral valve dynamics. Am Heart J 1972; 84: 141-144.

Cutler D J, Isner J M, Bracey A W, Hufnagel C A, Conrad P W, Roberts W C, Kerwin D M and Weintraub A M. Hemochromatosis heart disease: an unemphasized cause of potentially reversible restrictive cardiomyopathy. Am J Med 1980; 69: 923-928.

Dabestani A, Child J S, Henze E, Perloff J K, Schon H, Figueroa W G, Schelbert H R and Thessomboon S. Primary hemochromatosis: Anatomic and physiologic characteristics of the cardiac ventricles and their response to phlebotomy. Am J Cardiol 1984; 54: 153-160.

Davies M J. Pathology of Cardiac Valves. London: Butterworths 1980.

Davies M J. Invited review. The cardiomyopathies: a review of terminology, pathology and pathogenesis. Histopathology 1984; 8: 363-394.

Davies M J. The current status of myocardial disarray in hypertrophic cardiomyopathy. Br Heart J 1984; 51: 361-364.

Davies M J, Anderson R H and Becker A E. The Conduction System of the Heart. London: Butterworths 1983.

Davies M J, Fulton W F M and Robertson W B. The relation of coronary thrombosis to ischemic myocardial necrosis. J Pathol 1979; 127: 99-110.

Davies M J, Thomas T. The pathological basis and microanatomy of occlusive thrombus formation in human coronary arteries. Philosophical Transactions of the Royal Society of London 1981; 294: 225-229.

Davies M J, Thomas A C. Plaque fissuring – the cause of acute myocardial infarction, sudden ischemic death and crescendo angina. Br Heart J 1985; 53: 363-373.